Praise for *The Art of* ▊

"Dree has crafted an enchan▊
deeper connection with essen▊▊ ▊▊▊ ▊▊▊▊▊▊▊▊▊
through ritual and simple magickal practices like oils combined with tarot and pendulums for divination. Through reading this book, we can feel how alive and sacred the essential oils are and how they can be easily integrated into our daily magick.... You will discover what oils to buy and how to ethically source them, how to build powerful relationships with plant souls, how to use oils for magick, and so much more."

—**PAMELA CHEN**, author of *Enchanted Crystal Magic* and *The Mandarin Tree*

"This is more than a book about essential oils and aromatherapy—for me, this is a how-to guide on establishing a deep connection with the powerful essence of Mother Earth. Reading this book gave me a feeling like I was developing a personalized relationship with essential oils and the art of aromatherapy. By the end, I felt like I was in a deep, loving, magickal relationship....It is complete with exercises and recipes for the reader's experience, and a comprehensive index to reflect on later. This book is great for beginners, expansive for the intermediate worker, and a complementary reference for the well-practiced individual. This is a complete reference guide that belongs on every practitioner's bookshelf."

—**DR. JOY "GRANDDAUGHTER CROW" GRAY**, author of *Wisdom of the Natural World*

"The thoughtfulness and wisdom in *The Art of Aromatherapy in Magick* took me on a welcomed journey. Dree is genuinely hilarious and offers a generosity of wisdom and political thoughtfulness that weave together a truly holistic way to understand the science and magic of aromatherapy. Dree shares the practical facts while also leaving space for the reader to understand their own relationship to aromatherapy.... *The Art of Aromatherapy in Magick*'s unique take is a gift for seasoned witches, curious folks, and anyone seeking a deeper or renewed connection to aromatherapy. Take a deep breath and enjoy this magical ride."

—**SHARON PINK**, Portuguese and Polish, queer, femme, priestess, claircognizant witch

"*The Art of Aromatherapy in Magick* should not just be on every witch's bookshelf but in their hands, often! Never have I come across such a thorough book about how to use aromatherapy, and the way in which Dree links everything back to magickal practice makes this book an absolute must-read for any practicing witch or magickal practitioner. From how to shop ethically for your oils to making your own, creating blends, connecting more deeply with the wisdom and power of nature, this book contains everything you need to know to about enhancing your magickal practices, spells, and intentions with the support and guidance of our plant allies."

—**VICTORIA MAXWELL**, author, mentor, soul reader
& Kundalini yoga teacher

The
art
of
Aromatherapy
in
MAGICK

About the Author

Hailing from Vancouver Island, BC, Dree Amandi now calls Portland, OR, her home. Also known as "the Aroma Mystic," Dree considers herself a lifelong learner who is continually working toward mastering the art of spiritual aromatherapy to heal and harmonize. In 2022, Dree completed her ministerial training with Circle Sanctuary and was ordained as a Pagan Minister by Reverend Selena Fox. When not teaching workshops or engaged in community service, Dree can be found in her garden, on ocean shores, in the forest, and enjoying art and live music. Although Dree is awe-inspired by many things, her number one source of joy is the love she has for her family, particularly for her precious niblings Kiki and Kai-o Guy-o.

The
art
of
Aromatherapy
in
MAGICK
a guide for the
Modern Witch

Dree Amandi Pike

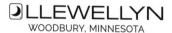
LLEWELLYN
WOODBURY, MINNESOTA

FIRST EDITION
First Printing, 2024

Cover design by Shannon McKuhen
Interior chakra figure on page 100 © Mary Ann Zapalac
Interior flower illustrations © Christine Lavdovsky
Interior pentacles on pages 67–68 by the Llewellyn Art Department

Llewellyn Publications is a registered trademark of Llewellyn
    Worldwide Ltd.

Library of Congress Cataloging-in-Publication Data (Pending)
ISBN: 978-0-7387-7003-1

Llewellyn Worldwide Ltd. does not participate in, endorse, or have any
authority or responsibility concerning private business transactions
between our authors and the public.

    All mail addressed to the author is forwarded but the publisher can-
not, unless specifically instructed by the author, give out an address or
phone number.

    Any internet references contained in this work are current at publica-
tion time, but the publisher cannot guarantee that a specific location
will continue to be maintained. Please refer to the publisher's website
for links to authors' websites and other sources.

Llewellyn Publications
A Division of Llewellyn Worldwide Ltd.
2143 Wooddale Drive
Woodbury, MN 55125-2989
www.llewellyn.com

Printed in the United States of America

Dedication

This book is dedicated to my friends and family who have significantly contributed to its manifestation through their loving support and relentless cheerleading. I must especially acknowledge my husband and wife who have supported me in more ways than I could ever put into words. Nathan, thank you for holding me up and supporting me through the daily struggle of writing this book. I literally couldn't have done it without you. Jade, since *before* day one of my spiritual journey, you have been there by my side. Thank you for always empowering me to show up as my fullest self.

Disclaimer

The material in this book is not intended as a substitute for trained medical or psychological advice. Readers are advised to consult their personal healthcare professionals regarding treatment of any illness or condition. The publisher and the author assume no liability for any injuries caused to the reader that may result from the reader's use of the content—whether herbal or otherwise—contained herein and recommend common sense when contemplating the practices described herein.

Contents

Introduction

Essential oils have a spirit and a purpose. Think about the alchemy involved in their formation. We are taking medicinal plant parts, drawing out their most beneficial elements, and isolating their most concentrated healing aspects. We are literally harvesting the very essence of the plant's existence. Do we have little plant souls bottled up in our cupboards? Yes, we do. But they aren't trapped like genies, they are ready and wanting to work for a cause. They are highly motivated, which is one of the reasons they're so inspiring to work with. They aren't bogged down or held back in any way; they are patiently waiting to be charged with intention and set forth to make change. Essential oils are not to be taken lightly; they are not to be wasted, dismissed, or ignored. If you have essential oils sitting in the back of a cupboard, go pull them out and use them. If you can't use them for whatever reason, give them to someone who can and will.

There are several good books out there that teach folks about various ways of rituals, rites, spellcraft, magick,

Pagan traditions, and spiritual paths. There are also several books that teach aromatherapy's global history, chemistry, research studies, medical applications, and essential oils in depth. This book was written for those seeking to use the tools of aromatherapy to enhance their magick and spiritual well-being. It was written for you, the spiritual practitioner. You, the essential oil enthusiast. You, the healer. You, the Witch. In fact, my approach to aromatherapy magick requires your unique individuality. That said, this book is written from my subjective perspective. The point of view, statements, suggestions, theology, and beliefs are based on my training and life experiences. My way is the right way for me alone. The goal is for you to discover the way that is right for you! I highly recommend getting yourself a journal so that you have a place to jot down your brilliant thoughts and creative ideas. Dedicated solely to your journey with aromatherapy and magick, your journal will serve as a record of knowledge gained and relationships built.

I have been a practicing Pagan since the early 1990s. My spiritual path began with solitary Wicca, and over the years it has grown and evolved in many ways within the Pagan sphere. I have been a Witch in solitude and in community, a student and an educator, deeply connected and slightly detached. My spirituality has ebbed and flowed always moving forward with Nature as my guide. Today, I identify as a Cio Amore Witch, and I follow an eclectic path. The Latin *cio* (pronounced chee-o) means to stir up, summon, or bring about. The Latin word *amore* (pronounced ah-more-eh) means love. As a Cio Amore Witch, I try to actively live by five key tenets: Lead with love, be sincere, do no harm, seek knowledge, and connect with nature. My Witchcraft is a love language, and my magick comes from a place of deep gratitude. It doesn't mean that I think everything is all sunshine and roses (that is simply not true), but it does mean that my magick most often intends to create or transform to help the world thrive, as opposed to stopping, blocking, or binding. I am not against others using those techniques in their magick; I just want you to understand who I am and how I work as you read.

I also have been working with essential oils and aromatherapy nearly as long as I've been Pagan, since about 1997. At that time, I worked for an aromatherapy company but didn't really combine my magickal practices with my aromatherapy practices for some years. I built a barrier separating my job from my spirituality that took me a while to dismantle. I was primarily using essential oils as a kind of medicine which, at that time, I defined as a healing treatment for the mind and body. When my definition of medicine started to include treatment for spiritual ailments, my world opened up: I started to study how essential oils, hydrosols, and carrier oils could promote whole healing of the mind, body, and spirit. And as a Witch, my studies needed to include magick.

My magick is based on the belief that everything is connected by universal energies. Scientifically, we know that all things in the universe are connected by physical energy because it can be objectively measured, thus requiring no faith or intuition. However, most people (spiritual or otherwise) agree that a metaphysical type of energy also exists that, although impossible to measure using the tools of science, can be profound and strongly felt. For me, the physical and metaphysical are intrinsically linked. That which exists as metaphysical can manifest as physical, and vice versa. Universal energies are infinite and transcendent; they mix and separate, flow around and through all things, transform and exchange. They are dynamic forces that exist in balance and neutrality and are at the foundation of all magick.

If we are all connected by energy, what we do can influence many other things, like ripples on a pond. Energetically existing as one and many is what enables us to make change within and outside of ourselves. Bringing about change through an act of magick requires deliberate intention and action from the practitioner working on both the physical and metaphysical planes. Acts of magick can appear in a million different ways, but my practice primarily uses meditation, visualization, divination, rites/ritual, body/energy work, shadow work/introspection, spellcraft, and communing with the Divine—all of which are perfectly complemented by essential oils and aromatherapy.

Like other ritual tools, essential oils respond to a practitioner's energy whether it's intentional or not, so it's important to treat them with love, care, and respect. They are wise, generous, and supportive, promoting wellness on every level. They enhance every spiritual path and experience, but when combined with magickal practice there is a particularly powerful synergy. The more you work with them in this way, the more inspired you will be.

The Art of Aromatherapy in Magick is your guide on how to think about the use of essential oils and carrier oils in a personal, customized, and mystical way. My approach uses the power behind real-time personal feedback—what I call the "subjective element"—and incorporates it into spiritual practices. Prioritizing the subjective element of aromatherapy when used for magick might be uncommon, but I hope this book challenges several commonly held beliefs by presenting thought-provoking ideas and innovative methodology. *The Art of Aromatherapy in Magick* will help you establish a personal tome of essential oils, develop relationships with them, create custom-tailored recipes informed by those relationships, and put those recipes to work enhancing your unique forms of magick. My heartfelt intention is for you to feel confident in spiritualizing and individualizing the tools and techniques of modern aromatherapy to create more profound, more meaningful, and more powerful magick. So, grab that journal and a pencil—let's dive in.

Chapter 1

Ancient Roots and Early Distillation

Long before chemical antiseptics, antibiotics, and pharmaceutical drugs, many cultures relied on the bactericidal, virucidal, and antiparasitic properties of medicinal aromatic plants (MAPs) to heal and protect them from illness. Aromatherapy's roots can be traced back to these ancient civilizations, where MAPs were used for medicinal *and* religious purposes. However, true essential oils must be extracted from MAPs by using steam distillation.

The process of steam distillation separates the volatile compounds (the essential oils) from the non-volatile components of plant matter. There is evidence that ancient Mesopotamia and ancient China both used rudimentary distillation apparatus as early as 6000 BCE, but ancient Egypt is one of the earliest civilizations we know to use steam distilled plant oils specifically for perfumes, incense, and phytopharmaceuticals. We can still see some of the aromatic recipes at the Temple of Horus at Edfu

(Behedet) inscribed on the walls more than two thousand years ago.[1] Around the same period, the Greek physician and botanist Pedanius Dioscorides (also known as the father of pharmacognosy), wrote extensively on methods of healing with MAPs in *De Materia Medica* or *On Medical Material*. This collection of medical texts and recipes references how one might extract, blend, and use plant oils for healing. One of the recommendations from *Materia Medica* is using bay leaf oil (*Laurus nobilis*) to warm the body and overcome exhaustion, among other things.[2]

The process of distillation was slowly refined over time, but it wasn't until early in the eleventh century that it was significantly improved. Persian physician Ibn Sīnā (Avicenna) advanced the distillation apparatus by adding a coiled cooling tube. This was a big technological leap forward that enabled him to pioneer a more precise and superior steam distillation technique. Following in his footsteps, Catalan physician Arnau de Vilanova refined the techniques enough to write the first true account essential oil extraction.[3] During the Renaissance, the German surgeon, alchemist, and botanist Hieronymus

1. Giacinto Bagetta, Marco Cosentino, and Tsukasa Sakurada, *Aromatherapy: Basic Mechanisms and Evidence Based Clinical Use* (CRC Press, 2015), 1.

2. Tess Anne Osbaldeston and Robert P. A. Wood, *Dioscorides: De Materia Medica: A New Indexed Version in Modern English* (IBIDIS Press, 2000), 46–47.

3. A. J. Rocke, "Agricola, Paracelsus, and 'Chymia'" *Ambix* vol. 32, no. 1 (1985): 38–45.

Brunschwig and others made further contributions to distillation technology. By the late fourteenth century, pharmacies were regularly steam distilling essential oils from plant matter to dispense as medicines.

Modern Aromatherapy

The term "aromatherapy" was coined by French chemist René-Maurice Gattefossé in the early twentieth century. He was inspired to study and work with the healing properties of essential oils after suffering a laboratory accident. His work, along with that of Dr. Jean Valnet, laid the foundation for modern aromatherapy and its integration with conventional medicine. Hospitals and wellness centers increasingly use essential oils for therapeutic benefits, particularly in stress relief and palliative care. Clinical research into the efficacy of aromatherapy has grown, providing a scientific basis for its use.

Our current understanding of how essential oils interact with our bodies tells us that nasal inhalation is the most effective way to deliver the oils' healing compounds to the brain and central nervous system. Nasal inhalation is also the most popular method of use and there are several tools to support the inhalation of essential oils, such as nebulizers, diffusers, and inhaler tubes. The second most common way to use essential oils is application to the skin. Often in conjunction with body treatments such as massage, lymph drainage, and compresses, topical application is the best way to deliver the oils' healing compounds to the organs and other body tissues. Absorption rates vary, but we know that the healing compounds of essential oils are small enough to penetrate our body's dermal layers and get absorbed into our microcirculation. From there, they can enter the body's main circulatory system and get transported around the entire body.

Aromatherapy in modern times is predominantly considered a tool for enhancing well-being with its myriad essential oils for relaxation, mood improvement, and physical ailments. Though deeply rooted in holistic wellness, contemporary practice often overlooks historical connections from times when ancient civilizations inextricably linked healing with spirituality and divinity. The burning of incense, the anointing of bodies with fragrant oils, and the use of aromatic herbs were not just for therapeutic purposes—they were integral to religious ceremonies, rituals, and the veneration of deities. This sacred aspect of aromatherapy highlights a profound reverence for the natural world and its deep connection to the spiritual realm. There is room for magick and divinity in our data-driven age; since the beginning of time, when humans began using medicinal aromatic plants, we who continue the practice have recognized that their use straddles the line between physical and metaphysical.

Bridging Science and Magick

Most likely, you have heard of the ancient Greek theory of the four basic elements: earth, air, fire, and water. For two thousand years, these elements were thought to be the building blocks that made up all matter. This theory was supported by philosophers, physicians, and scientists until Aristotle questioned whether the four elements could make up the planets and stars. He observed that the planets and stars were unchanging, in contrast to the mutable and terrestrial four elements. He reasoned that there must in fact be a fifth element: aether, a celestial substance that made up the heavens. Others adopted his new theory, and the diverse polytheistic population asserted that the fifth element must be an essence that filled the cosmos, a pure essence of life that the gods breathe like air. People believed that the fifth element was necessary for any type of matter to exist, and furthermore, it could cure all disease if it was somehow isolated. As a spiritual practitioner and aromatherapist, this concept really resonates with me. I too believe that essential oils are tangible expressions of life force that bridge the gap between the mundane and the Divine. During the medieval period, Aristotle's writings were translated and re-copied, at which time it took on a new name in Latin, *quinta essentia,* from which we derive our word "quintessence" and the term "essential oil."[4]

Sacred Keys

Aromatherapy can improve our whole wellness, providing healing to all aspects of our being. The restorative power of essential oils usher us toward physical, emotional, and spiritual health. Drawn from nature, essential oils are charged with the raw energy of the Universe, acting as links to the divine forces that govern our planet and beyond. They allow us to attune ourselves to these cosmic forces, allowing us to feel the interconnectedness of all life and existence.

Each essential oil possesses a unique energy that vibrates in our presence, harmonizing with our own energy to bring about a state of equilibrium. They are like sacred keys that unlock the doors to our inner workings. When we tap into these hidden layers, we can initiate profound internal transformations that reflect externally in our everyday lives. For example, the oil of lavender is associated with tranquility, helping to alleviate anxiety and promote a sense of peace and relaxation. When diffused in the home or applied topically, it serves to not only transform our environment into a haven of serenity but also to quiet the mind and prepare us for introspection, meditation, and spiritual practice. On the other hand, oils such as euca-

4. Gerard Watson, *Philosophical Studies: Aristotle's Concept of Matter* 20, iss. 0, 175–84. Maynooth 1971.

lyptus and rosemary are invigorating and energizing. They can cleanse negative energy and promote a fresh, positive perspective.

Remember, these divine substances are not just tools of healing, they are the catalysts of our transformation. They possess the power to bring about needed changes in our lives, acting as our guides on the path of self-discovery and spiritual evolution. When we incorporate them into our spiritual lives, we invoke their wisdom and power, harnessing their energy to heal, inspire, and transcend.

When I am doing any type of magick, I feel it in the deepest parts of my being—I get goosebumps and full body shivers. That's when I know I am tapped into the fabric of the Universe, the Source energy, the Quinta Essentia. Calling on an essential oil in these moments is profound. The oils radiate a feeling of delighted eagerness, ready to fulfill their healing purpose as they have done for thousands of years. It is an honor to work with them in a magickal way. The more I do, the more deeply I understand that the combined potential of aromatherapy and magick is limitless.

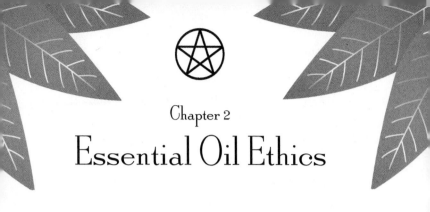

Chapter 2

Essential Oil Ethics

These days, there is a lot of visibility around essential oils. They are available in all types of major retail outfits and are commonly used in both medicinal and non-medicinal ways. They feel familiar and approachable even to people who are not usually interested in alternative modalities of healing. If we're being honest, most of us start getting into essential oils simply because they smell good, they are easy to find, and they can replace some toxic household cleaners. While all those things are true, it doesn't take long for us to notice that the more we use them, the more we want to use them in different ways, including healing of the mind, body, and spirit. And although we are so fortunate to have easy access to essential oils to experiment with, the hard truth is that these plant essences are often created for us at great cost. For context, let's look at what essential oils are and where they come from.

What Is an Essential Oil?

Surprisingly, essential oils are not actually oils—they're complex concentrations of water-insoluble and volatile chemical compounds that exist within most plants. These compounds aren't necessarily required for the plants to live, but they do have many functions that help them thrive. Among other things, essential oils can attract pollinators, repel predators, and be emitted as chemical signals to enable communication.

Essential oils are not necessarily in all plant parts, and a few plants can produce more than one type of essential oil, depending on which part is processed. For example, the generous bitter orange plant (*Citrus aurantium*) provides us with neroli oil from its flowers, petitgrain oil from its leaves, and orange oil from the peel of its fruit. Depending on the plant, essential oils can be extracted from rhizomes or roots, stems or wood, resin, gum, bark, twigs, grass, leaves, needles, flowers, fruit, seeds, or peels. The majority of essential oils are extracted from plant matter that goes through the steam distillation process. Aside from a few exceptions such as the expression of citrus peels, steam distillation is the only way to produce true essential oils.

Steam distillation requires a closed system of equipment that captures and directs steam from boiling water. Steam is forced through plant matter and draws out the essential oil, thereby infusing the steam. That steam is then cooled, which causes it to condense into a liquid form. Because essential oils are not water soluble, the condensation process separates the liquid into two. The highly valued essential oil sits atop the water byproduct and gets skimmed off for bottling. The water byproduct, called hydrosol, does not contain essential oils but does contain the plant's water-soluble elements both aromatic and therapeutic. It is often bottled and sold as floral water or simply disposed of. Theoretically, anyone with the right equipment and training could distill essential oils for themselves on a small scale. However, to get a little bit of essential oil requires a lot of plant matter, and the ratio makes do-it-yourself steam distillation unrealistic for most people. Large-scale production for the essential oil consumer goods market gives us access to oils and hydrosols that would otherwise be virtually impossible to obtain but unfortunately leaves a pretty ugly footprint.

Big Business

As a professional aromatherapist, I am somewhat complicit in the many harms caused by commercial industry of essential oil production, but as a Pagan I am motivated to try to do better by our living planet. I have the honor and obligation to learn what I can to make informed decisions that make sense for me as an individual while also being mindful and considerate of others. By making intentional choices guided by my personal ethics, I can have some hope that my work with these divine essences will do much more good than harm. After all, they are universal healers that should be cherished, used, and celebrated. With that said, I'm about to become aromatherapy's biggest party pooper.

At the time of this writing, an approximate market value of essential oils in the US alone is more than 3.5 *billion* dollars. That means the market demand from the United States alone was more than 187,392,923 pounds of essential oils per year. Of course, the vast majority of essential oil demand is not coming from those who use them to heal, do magick, or make a nice household cleaner. Most of the demand comes from the food and beverage industry, which uses essential oils in flavoring, followed by cosmetic and fragrance industries.

As consumers, it is important for us to know what our dollars are supporting. Although some artisan distillers have made it their top priority to reduce the footprint of their essential oils, there is no avoiding the fact that they are resource intensive. On average, producing essential oils on a large commercial scale has proven to be damaging in several ways, including environmentally, ecologically, and culturally. My intention here is not to shame, or guilt, or overwhelm. There is no judgment or pressure here, because we all have our own shade of green; this is just about learning. When we ask challenging questions, the answers might feel uncomfortable, but when we use all the uncovered information to define ethical deal-breakers, we can make better choices and uphold the values that are important to us. Take a breath; we're going to unpack this a little bit.

Commercial Farming

Most plants that are grown for essential oil production are cultivated in huge commercial farms, which mean fewer indigenous plants, fewer wild insect and animal habitats, less biodiversity, and ever-weakening soil. Depending on where the farms are built, it could even mean that forest was clear-cut to make space for the crops. Big agriculture needs to reduce the risk of losing their living investment, which often means the heavy use of water for irrigation, fertilizers, pesticides, and sometimes herbicides. If the farm is in a place with incompatible weather patterns, it will need artificial climate control measures, which use a lot of energy to heat, cool, and provide lights to stimulate growth.

Once the cultivated plant matter is mature and harvested, it needs to get to the distillers. This means transportation on container ships, trains, planes, and commercial trucks, all of which consume a lot of fuel and emit a lot of exhaust. The distiller steam distills the plant matter in a process that uses significant amounts of water and amounts of energy to heat and cool it, at the very least. When the essential oils are ready for bottling, the carbon footprint of bottle manufacturing and the eventual disposal of the plastic and glass add to the overall footprint of essential oil production. The bottles are packed in boxes usually made of either recycled paper, pine tree pulp, or a combination of both, which adds another manufacturing and waste footprint. When ready for market, the boxes of bottles are again transported by vehicles of mass pollution until they eventually find their way to our homes. Take another deep breath.

Wild Harvesting

Some of the problems with commercially farmed oil-bearing plants can be solved or mitigated by wild harvesting. To qualify as wild-harvested, the essential oil-bearing plants must be grown in their native habitats, harvested in a sustainable way, and even though they usually can't be certified as organic (a separate process), in theory they should all be growing in organic conditions. The most obvious question here is: how do we know if these rules are actually being followed? The discouraging answer is that we often don't.

Third-party certification auditors can be brought in to verify that growing conditions are noninvasive and the harvesting done sustainably and ethically, but that verification is not a requirement of any company. The auditors need to be hired by the company that wants to be audited. If it is found that the plant species they harvested weren't grown in a farmed environment, they can still label their essential oils as wild-harvested. There isn't a governing body that oversees this practice, nor are there consistent rules or requirements for enforcement. Unfortunately, there are many threatened and protected plant species that are being wild-harvested even though they are headed to extinction. You read that right—even though this method is marketed as being a greener option, some bottles of essential oils labeled as wild-harvested could just as rightfully be labeled as poached, smuggled, and illegally sold. Breathe in, breathe out.

Defining Deal-Breakers

There isn't anything humanmade that is without some level of cost, environmental, ecological, cultural, or other. We still choose to use them because the benefits outweigh the costs. For example, I buy toilet paper, but if it is made from the wood pulp of clear-cut virgin forests, that's a deal-breaker. It's the same with the oils: if they were distilled from plant matter grown with pesticides, that's a deal-breaker.

Deal-breakers are intended to inspire meaningful but attainable changes to improve the ways we exist in the world. They don't need to be extreme to make a positive difference in the world; it's all about finding the balance that's right for each of us as individuals. Maybe it's doable for a person to only buy small-batch distilled essential oils from locally sourced and sustainably harvested indigenous plants grown within a hundred miles of their home. Fabulous! Maybe it's only doable for a person to exclusively buy essential oils labeled as organic. Fabulous! There aren't any wrong choices when it comes to deciding how we are going to be better citizens of our planet. Ask yourself: what are your most important considerations? Are your ethical essential oil deal-breakers environmental? Ecological? Cultural? And what are the comparable alternatives? Are those options better or worse?

Helpful Resources

For a long time, I primarily relied on the following two sources of information to help me define and stay within the boundaries of my personal deal-breakers–CITES and IUCN. The Convention on International Trade in Endangered Species of Wild Fauna and Flora (CITES) is an international treaty agreement that ensures that the survival of wild animal and plant species isn't threatened by trade. CITES provides participating governments with criteria and certification for the ethical trade of biological imports and exports.

The International Union for Conservation of Nature (IUCN) is a global environmental organization that has both a massive conservationist network and species database that generates what's known as the "Red List." The IUCN Red List provides the conservation status on thousands of biological species using their seven-category scale starting with "Least Concern" and progressing to the final category, "Extinct." By simply searching their botanical names, I can use the IUCN database tool to get the worldwide conservation status of my essential oils' plants, plus any I am considering purchasing. The information that these organizations provide is invaluable, but navigating their websites and reviewing their data can be intimidating and time consuming.

Lucky for us, a nonprofit organization committed to advancing global education, research, and the sustainable stewardship of medicinal and aromatic plants was founded in 2017 by Dr. Kelly Ablard—the Airmid Institute.

Before Airmid Institute, I would spend countless frustrating hours sifting through information trying to find comprehensive and up to date content that only pertained to the ethics of essential oils. I would compile my own lists using the data I gathered from up to five different organizations and take notes on ethical considerations prompted by various articles and papers.

Of course, it was time well spent, but thanks to Dr. Kelly Ablard and the Airmid Institute, a large portion of that time has been given back to me. I am not exaggerating when I tell you that this nonprofit organization changed my life, not to mention all the positive changes they have made all over our planet by protecting oil-bearing species and the communities that are connected to them.

On their user-friendly website, these generous geniuses offer a lot of the information that I need, and none of the convoluting information that I don't need. They even maintain a list of threatened, near threatened, and CITES-protected species used in aromatherapy, perfumery, and aromatic herbalism. Here's the best part, this list is updated and emailed out to members every six months! Honestly, if I had to choose one take away from this chapter, it would be for everyone to become a member of the Airmid Institute. I have endless gratitude and respect for their work and if this is the first time you are learning about them, you're welcome.

Quality Over Quantity

Another factor to consider is an oil's quality. Details matter in aromatherapy and magick, and we should strive for the highest quality of both. Several factors affect essential oil quality, including the time of day the plants are harvested, the temperatures reached in the distillation process, and what stage of development the plant parts were in at the time of harvesting. For instance, when older leaves of sage (*Salvia officinalis*) plants are used to extract essential oil, the oil can have high levels of α-thujone which could cause neurotoxicity or may even be carcinogenic when used over a long period of time. However, essential oil extracted from young sage leaves has very low amounts of α-thujone, making it safe to use over long periods. We can only gather this kind of information from the essential oil's distiller. Most reputable distillers have this information and more readily available on their websites. By taking the time to research the details of how a distiller harvests and processes plant matter, we can ensure that we are purchasing the highest quality. We want fresh essential oils made from premium plant parts harvested at peak times and distilled at optimal temperatures. Especially as it relates to safety, we do not need many essential oils, but we do need the best.

Pricing

As we are analyzing quality, remember that a higher price does not always mean a better product. The pricing of essential oils should generally reflect how much it costs to produce, but just as with any other consumer product, prices are sometimes inflated to increase profit margins. The range of prices across essential oil varieties is massive, depending on how easily it can be extracted. Some essential oils are easy to coax out, making them inexpensive, and others can cost more than $20,000 per pound. For example, it takes about 10,000 pounds of rose petals to distill one pound of rose essential oil (*Rosa damascena*). To be clear, that is 5 tons of plant matter for 1 pound of essential oil. It makes sense that it costs around $270 for a 5 mL bottle of rose essential oil, compared to the $5 it costs to buy the same amount of sweet orange essential oil (*Citrus sinensis*). One might look at the price differential and think that rose oil is more precious, but I choose to value all my essential oils based on the potential of their power. In other words, while they may not be of the same monetary value, I consider rose and sweet orange essential oil to be equally valuable in practice. They are unique and equally important in terms of what they can offer my magickal work.

Examining Bottle Labels

Wherever profit is involved, there are people who will do whatever it takes to make more, more, more. There are many unscrupulous essential oil companies that increase their profits by taking advantage of their customers' trust. One of the easiest scams for them to execute is to lower their cost of essential oils by diluting them with natural or synthetic components and selling them at full price.

Unethical essential oil companies often get away with using a tactic of ambiguous labeling. This is a tricky strategy that aims to deliberately confuse the customer by adding information that is misleading and omitting information that is clarifying. For example, by intentionally leaving out the Latin botanical name on a bottle of "100% pure lavender essential oil," one could legally sell a less expensive variety of *Lavendula* at the price of the most expensive variety. Alternatively, a seller could substitute descriptive language with marketing language to confuse the customer. For example, by marketing a bottle as "100% therapeutic grade lavender oil," one could take an inexpensive base oil, add only a small percentage of lavender essential oil, imply that it was 100 percent pure essential oil and legally sell it. Thankfully, most countries have labeling laws that aim to prevent unscrupulous companies from making false claims. If we know what should be on an essential oil label, we can better protect ourselves.

When working with essential oils, the goal is to get high-quality, small footprint, unadulterated products. For most, the label can provide more than adequate amounts of information to discern whether a particular bottle of essential oil fits within their ethos.

Quality Assessment

When assessing the quality of an essential oil from its label, look for:

- The Latin botanical name to ensure you are getting the species that you want
- Organic certification—although not always possible, it's definitely preferable
- Geographical origin of the plant matter, which directly affects the quality of essential oil
- The specific plant parts that were distilled; you only want oil from the premium parts
- The method of extraction to ensure it is either steam distilled or cold expressed
- The date of manufacture or expiration because essential oils eventually oxidize
- A batch lot number for traceability, and so you can ask for its gas chromatography-mass spectrometry

(GCMS) analysis results. This test identifies all the constituents that make up an essential oil so its purity and authenticity may be verified.

- The name and location of the distiller so that you can research the source of their plant matter, where it was grown, and how that might affect the oil quality. You may also want to be able to contact them with questions.

Footprint Assessment

When assessing the footprint of an essential oil from its label, look for:

- The Latin botanical name along with the origin of its plant matter to cross reference with lists of threatened species
- Any organic certification to assess potential negative environmental impact
- The origin of the plant matter to research potential negative cultural and social impact
- A CITES certification to ensure that it wasn't illegally traded
- The name and location of the distiller so that you can research their ethical sourcing standards and contact them with questions

Purity Assessment

When assessing the purity of an essential oil from its label, look for:

- The Latin botanical name to ensure that it is exactly the variety you want
- Organic certification to ensure that there are no chemical contaminants
- A statement that explicitly states "100% pure essential oil"; it's illegal to make blatantly false claims
- A batch lot number for traceability and so you can ask for its gas chromatography-mass spectrometry (GCMS) analysis results should you want to see its chemical breakdown
- The name and location of the distiller so that you can research their production/quality control standards and contact them with questions

Making Informed Decisions

It is not easy to face hard truths and hidden costs, which is why many people don't inquire about quality standards and ethical sourcing. But you are brave, smart, and mindful. Ask the questions, seek the answers, and use your knowledge to make informed decisions that will support the things that you value most.

If you discover that an essential oil in your collection has qualities that now make it a deal-breaker, use it with gratitude and joy—and then don't re-buy it. As we continue to learn and evolve, our ideals shift and we need to adjust how we manage our deal-breakers, not to mention the dynamics of sourcing and changes in status of oil-bearing plants around the world. Always choose quality over quantity. Only buy the essential oils that you need, and honor them by using them in beautiful ways.

I need to acknowledge the elephant in the room: I mentioned that we do not need many essential oils, but I definitely have a lot. I use them to heal, transform, and empower, but ultimately no one *needs* essential oils. The ways in which they can improve our lives are countless, but we really don't *need* them at all. I like to remind myself of that fact every so often, and it's important to mention it here. With all the privilege and excess in this country, it's easy to take things for granted. I don't want to lose sight of the fact that regardless of their monetary worth and perceived value, essential oils are utterly precious on their own.

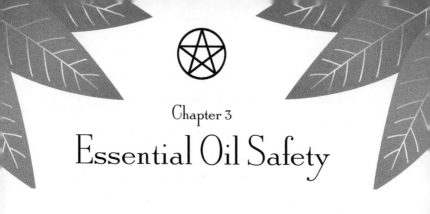

Essential Oil Safety

One of the most important things to consider when working with essential oils is safety. They seem innocent enough, but essential oils are highly concentrated and can be dangerous and damaging to the skin and internal organs if used incorrectly. Just like any other potentially hazardous endeavor, do your research using multiple sources of reliable information before starting. Educating yourself about the safety and proper use of essential oils is key to enjoying their many benefits. These potent and powerful products should be used with humble respect and caution.

Proper Storage

The amount of time that an oil is usable largely depends on its exposure to heat, light, and air. All of which should be avoided to extend the life of any oil, so store your bottles of oil in a cool dark place that is easy to access. Despite all our efforts to keep our oils from degrading, all oils will eventually oxidize and expire. Every time you use your oils, take a glance at their expiration dates. It's a good habit that will help to keep your collection fresh.

Essential Oil Toxicity

Essential oils are rapidly absorbed into our body systems, which is one of their strengths as a healing modality. However, the other side of that coin is that it is possible to overwhelm the body if too much is introduced into its system at once. Long exposure to active diffusion, ingestion, and topical applications using unsafe dilution ratios increases the risk of essential oil toxicity. The range of symptoms associated with essential oil toxicity is broad, making it sometimes difficult to diagnose. Symptoms include (but are not limited to) headaches, sore throat, drowsiness, shortness of breath, coughing, gagging or choking, nausea, vomiting, and diarrhea. I have never experienced toxicity directly, but I do know of three separate accounts of essential oil toxicity from people leaving their active diffusers on 24/7. Thankfully, the solution was easy: they just needed to stop constantly diffusing essential oils and start breathing fresh air. To reduce your chances of toxicity reactions, limit your use of an active diffuser to a maximum of ninety minutes per day, thirty minutes being ideal.

Skin Irritations

Before using a new essential oil on the skin, I recommend performing a patch test by diluting it in a carrier and applying it to a small area of skin. Be aware of potential skin irritation or allergic reactions and if any redness, itching, or burning occurs after 24 hours, discontinue use.

It's always very important to dilute your essential oils in a carrier, a rule that applies to all essential oils, in my opinion. I even dilute lavender (*Lavandula angustifolia*) and tea tree (*Melaleuca alternifolia*), which are commonly used directly on the skin, or "neat." Unscented lotion, hair conditioner, and castile soap are great carrier options: they blend well with essential oils and if they separate, are easy to mix with a good shake.

Essential oils and water don't mix, so when you aren't diluting with an oil-based carrier such as lotion or carrier oil, you need to use a dispersant. Using products like Solubol, polysorbate 20, or greater than 70 percent alcohol will help disperse essential oils into water, diluting them to a safe level for skin contact. When making dry products such as oil-free bath salts, bath powder, and dry shampoo, I use Natrasorb, a modified arrowroot starch made from cassava root. It is hard to beat this cosmetic ingredient because it's specifically designed to capture and hold essential oils, making them safe for skin contact in a powder form. Always check the manufacturer recommended blending ratio of dispersant to essential oil. Generally speaking, Solubol is 4:1 and polysorbate 20 is 1:1.

Sunlight Exposure

An important yet often-overlooked safety consideration is how the skin reacts to a topically applied essential oil when exposed to sunlight. When using essential oils on the skin, it's important to be aware of the phototoxicity and photosensitizing risk. Some essential oils will chemically burn the skin when exposed to UV rays. I have definitely taken this risk lightly in the past. One time I applied some properly diluted bergamot essential oil to the back of my neck to help me relax before bedtime. The next day, I went outside on a moderately sunny day and ended up with a chemical burn of blisters and welts. To be extra careful, I no longer use potentially phototoxic essential oils at all on hands, faces, necks, temples, and ears. In the summer, I won't use them at all.

Cold-expressed citrus essential oils are notoriously important to watch. Interestingly, steam distilled citrus essential oils don't seem to react on the skin in the same way when exposed to UV light, because their chemical makeup is changed during the steam distillation process. The primary offenders are in a class of phytochemicals called furanocoumarins. Thankfully, it is possible to buy essential oils that have been deliberately and specifically altered to remove the offending furanocoumarins, most commonly bergaptene, psoralens, and oxypeucedanin.

Medical Considerations

Each essential oil has the potential to make physical and metaphysical change, which is really what their healing and magickal benefits boil down to. However, a healing change in one person's body can be a harmful change in another person's body. For example, if I have low blood pressure, I don't want to use a lot of essential oils that might lower it further. But if I have high blood pressure, I might want to use the essential oils that will lower it on a consistent basis. In our attempts to support total wellness of mind, body, and spirit, let's not exacerbate any underlying medical conditions. It's critically important to educate yourself on possible health contraindications of essential oil use.

Regarding food allergies, sometimes we won't have the same reaction to an essential oil that we might have an allergic reaction to if we ate the oil's origin plant. But why gamble? If I had a food allergy, I wouldn't use the essential oil that was distilled from it. There are so many other amazing options to choose from, it's just not worth the risk. Ingesting essential oils or using them internally shouldn't be done without close guidance from a qualified and experienced professional aromatherapist. Essential oils are not the same as food; they are digested, absorbed, and metabolized very differently. If you want to absorb the medicinal benefits from plants through ingestion, seek a qualified herbalist.

Folks at Higher Risk

Some folks are at a higher risk of experiencing negative side effects. Symptoms of epilepsy and asthma can be aggravated with essential oil use. Theoretically, any oil could be problematic for those with these conditions, so I recommend consulting a professional aromatherapist to decrease your level of risk.

I do not recommend using essential oils with kids under twelve, but I tend to err heavily on the side of caution. Of course, there are several essential oils that can be used to treat children and infants, and working with a professional aromatherapist can help navigate safe usage. People who are pregnant can be at higher risk when using essential oils, and some could harm a fetus depending on its stage of gestation. If the goal is to carry the pregnancy to full term, it is ill-advised to use essential oils that might affect hormone levels or stimulate any kind of uterine activity. This is particularly important early in the first trimester and into the second.

Professional Help

My opinion on the benefits of working with a professional aromatherapist is definitely biased. Not because I am one, but because I know what they can offer. I find that most people have heard about aromatherapists but are unclear about what we do, what training we have, and if we are monitored by a governing body. Hopefully, this chapter will help answer the question "why should I work with a professional?"

Degrees and Certifications

Professional aromatherapists are unregulated in the United States. However, professional aromatherapists in the US generally seek certification from the National Association for Holistic Aromatherapy (NAHA). This nonprofit organization is as close as it gets to a regulating body for this industry and can provide some credibility and accountability for aromatherapists. They promote and uphold high standards of practice, compliance with safety standards, commitment to their code of ethics, consistent standards for aromatherapy schools, a high level of aromatherapy education from a NAHA-merited school, and continuing education credits (CEs). Here is a summary of the educational requirements for the three levels of NAHA certification.

Level 1: Aromatherapist

To graduate, students must complete fifty hours of aromatherapy education from a NAHA-approved school. Prerequisites for these programs include:

- Completion of a first-year Anatomy & Physiology undergraduate class from an accredited institution. Typically, this class covers body tissues and the integumentary system, joints and the skeletal system, muscle tissue and the muscular system, nervous tissue and the central nervous system, the peripheral nervous system, the autonomic nervous system, the endocrine system, cellular structure and cell types, and basic chemistry.

Graduates must complete five hours of NAHA-approved continuing education credits (CEs) per year to maintain their certification status.

Level 2: Professional Aromatherapist

To graduate, students must complete 150 hours of aromatherapy education from an approved school in addition to the following prerequisites:

- NAHA Level 1 Aromatherapist certification.
- Completion of a second-year Anatomy & Physiology undergraduate class. Typically, this class covers the reproductive system, the cardiovascular system, the lymphatic system, the immune system, the urinary system, and the digestive system.

Graduates must complete ten hours of NAHA-approved CEs per year to maintain certification status.

Level 3: Clinical Aromatherapist

To graduate, students must complete 100 hours of aromatherapy education from an approved school in addition to the following prerequisites:

- A minimum of one year of direct clinical aromatherapy experience.
- NAHA Level 2 Professional Aromatherapist certification.
- Completion of a graduate level class in Advanced Pathophysiology. Typically, this class advances knowledge of anatomy and physiology, explaining the mechanisms of diseases and pathophysiological conditions that affect the integumentary system, the circulatory system, the reproductive system, the musculoskeletal system, the lymphatic and immune system, the endocrine system, the nervous system, the urinary system, and the digestive system.

Graduates must complete fifteen hours of NAHA-approved CEs per year to maintain certification status.

Finding an Aromatherapist

I highly recommend seeking out help from aromatherapists who are NAHA-certified, although I'm sure there are amazing aromatherapists out there who aren't. Since I have been through the certification process and know what it takes to graduate, I feel more comfortable using it as a baseline to assess knowledge and experience levels.

Every professional aromatherapy practice looks a bit different depending on the practitioner. Any can offer clients general consulting, essential oil recommendations, and basic custom blending, but many of us specialize, focusing our services within our niche. It's worth contacting a few different professionals to ask questions that will help determine if they are a good match for you personally. For instance, I specialize in spiritual aromatherapy; although I can offer other services, I will usually only accept clients who are specifically seeking me for support to incorporate aromatherapy into a spiritual aspect of their lives. If that is what you need, I'm your pro! However, I am also a Witch, so I am not a great match for some. I also won't work with several oils due to my ethical deal-breakers. That itself might be problematic for some, too. Maybe my sense of humor is too weird, maybe my swearing is offensive, maybe I don't see clients early enough in the day. Any information that might affect the relationship between you and your practitioner should be sought out up front. Don't be afraid to get answers for what matters to you.

For some reason, what I'm about to share isn't well known or widely discussed, but everyone needs to know this incredibly useful information because it's a game-changer—it will increase your essential oil knowledge, decrease waste and superfluous collections, and make magickal aromatherapy more effective. Once you've established a relationship with a professional aromatherapist, they'll be able to sell you high quality essential oils by the drop. Why is this a game-changer? You'll gain access to a huge collection of essential oils, you'll no longer need to have a collection from which you only ever need a couple drops, and you can test for sensitivity before committing to buying or using full-sized bottles. It's more likely you'll experiment and play with what works best in any given magickal work when the barrier to entry is lower."

Isn't it exciting to think about the possibilities? For this reason alone, working with a professional can make the journey into aromatherapy much safer, faster, and more affordable. The best advice I can offer is to find a qualified and experienced, professional spiritual aromatherapist who specializes in the magickal uses of essential oils. They are absolutely worth the investment, and so are you.

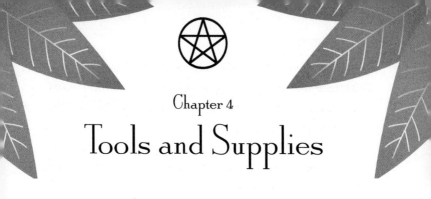

Chapter 4

Tools and Supplies

With the right tools, you can start your journey into magickal aromatherapy with confidence. In addition to your essential oils, you'll need a journal, bottles, droppers, carrier oils, a small liquid measure, and a diffuser. Naturally, there are a million other cool things that are great to have, but this is all that you really need.

Dedicated Grimoire

Get a blank journal and start documenting your journey with aromatherapy and magick. Trust me, it will become your go-to resource as you work through this book. There will be several opportunities to develop a powerful tome of information, observations, and experiences unique to you and your personal journey of growth, and it will become richer with every entry. In my opinion, a grimoire (as opposed to a journal) has a purposeful energy of spiritual transformation, evolving it from a quick reference of essential oil profiles to a magickal tool.

If nothing else, it's worth developing your grimoire to ensure you have a good record of your recipes and witchcraft. I cannot stress this enough: write down as much as you can with your recipes. I've created many amazingly powerful recipes that I have never been able to duplicate, and it is beyond annoying when a need arises for a recipe that I forgot to document.

Here's an example of what a grimoire recipe might include:

- Who the recipe was made for
- Why it was needed
- The magickal intention
- The date, including day of the week, and time
- The moon phase
- The geographic location
- Any noteworthy events or other info: weather, meteor showers, frogs loudly singing all around you—whatever seems significant and unique to that moment
- The method of aromatherapy application and why
- The essential oils, hydrosols, and/or carrier oils used and why
- The spiritual/magickal practice(s) involved and why
- Magickal tools used and why

- Words used, invocations made, divine beings present
- Any unexpected things that occurred

You may not think you'll need all this information again, but if you don't write it down, you definitely will. In times of impromptu magick, I'll just jot down critical information—the magick's intention, the date, the time, and the aromatherapy used. Later, in a less spontaneous moment, I will transfer the recipe into my grimoire with any other information I think is important to note. Hopefully, I remember all of it. Being able to look back at all these magickal details is probably my favorite thing about having a grimoire. It can hold many beautiful memories that can retell the story of your spirituality, humanity, and divinity.

Bottles

Glass bottles are necessary for storing essential oils in a safe manner. If stored in plastic, your essential oils may get contaminated by leaching chemicals. Most commonly, when we buy essential oils, they come in dark glass bottles that hold 5 milliliter (mL) or 10 mL quantities. The glass needs to be a dark color or opaque to protect the essential oils from light, which will degrade them. I like to have clean 5 mL, 10 mL, and 30 mL bottles ready for my blends. I also like to have 30 mL and 50 mL jars on hand for things like scrubs and creams. I make sure to have reducer tops, roller-ball tops, and mister spray tops available to increase the options for how I might want to want to use my blends.

Aromatherapy supply shops, apothecary shops, crafting stores, and online retailers have many options. I suggest purchasing bottles that all have the same sized threaded opening. This will make all your lid options and bottle sizes interchangeable. Aromatherapy bottle openings are small, so a funnel will help prevent spills when you're filling them. Remember to label your bottles and include the closest expiration date of the bottle's contents.

Droppers

Droppers are needed to measure and distribute essential oils in small amounts. Although professionals sometimes measure by weight, DIY aromatherapy recipes most often measure by the drop. Some people use single-use plastic pipettes, but I prefer a good ol' fashioned glass dropper with a squeeze bulb. Using a glass dropper ensures that my oils won't get contaminated from leaching plastic, and I can clean them out and reuse them. Always use a clean dropper when transferring essential oils from their original bottles to avoid cross contamination. I keep mine clean and reusable by washing them out with warm water and dish soap, then air drying. These droppers can usually be purchased wherever aromatherapy bottles are sold as well as in the first-aid section of most drug stores.

Carrier Oils

These are absolutely essential for the topical application of any essential oils. The number one reason is for safety, yes, but they also serve as a solid foundation for the intention in your magickal aromatherapy practices. Chapter 10 covers carrier oil options in more detail, but here are a couple of favorites to get you started.

A lot of my aromatherapy magick is rooted in empowerment, abundance, and fertility. Because of what they add to my work energetically and physically, sunflower oil, grapeseed oil, and avocado oil are my go-to carrier oils. The most commonly used carriers in professional aromatherapy are jojoba oil and fractionated coconut oil because they are odorless, lovely on the skin, and have a long shelf life. As you become more proficient, I recommend experimenting a bit with oils you might already have in your kitchen. Don't be afraid to try carrier oils that already have an aroma. Blending essential oils with carrier oils that already smell yummy, such as sesame oil, is a fun challenge.

Liquid Measures

Measuring liquids is an important part of blending. Recommended ratios between essential oils and carriers are specific, and ignoring them can be unsafe. A small glass measuring cup or beaker marked with milliliters works best, but you could use a teaspoon (~5 mL) and a tablespoon (~15 mL) for measuring out most recipes. Here are my most used dilutions:

- 5% essential oil blend =
  10 mL carrier oil + 10 drops essential oil
- 3% essential oil blend =
  10 mL carrier oil + 6 drops essential oil
- 1% essential oil blend =
  10 mL carrier oil + 2 drops essential oil

Just like your bottles and droppers, keep your measuring tools clean to prevent cross contamination.

Diffusers

Diffusers come in several types, including heat diffusers, ultrasonic, nebulizers, passive diffusers, and nasal inhaler tubes. They are all a key part of aromatherapy equipment. Each type has its own benefits, so it is helpful to consider the type of magick you're doing before selecting one.

Active Diffusers

In the context of aromatherapy, more is not better, particularly when using an active diffuser. When using this type of diffuser, limit the length of time it disperses essential oil into your environment. Too much can cause some negative side effects, including essential oil toxicity. I usually limit my active diffuser usage to thirty minutes per twenty-four-hour period. When I have need for more time using an active diffuser, I do ninety minutes per forty-eight hours maximum, very rarely needing more than that.

Heat diffusers obviously use heat to vaporize essential oils, creating a powerful aroma charged with active and warm energy. This kind of diffuser can be particularly helpful when doing any kind of hearth or kitchen magick. My favorite type of heat diffuser is a ceramic tealight oil burner. With this type of diffuser, all the elements are represented: earth as the pottery, air as the evaporating vapor, fire as the candle flame, water in the burner reservoir, and spirit represented by the essential oils. They are perfect for altars and daily devotion rituals.

Ultrasonic diffusers are a good choice for creating sacred spaces because they use water with essential oils to create a fine mist that can quickly fill a room with scent.

Nebulizing diffusers disperse essential oils without using any extra liquids or heat, allowing the essential oil to fully retain its therapeutic properties, which makes them ideal for meditation magick.

Inhalers are portable hand-held devices that allow the scent of essential oils to be inhaled directly from the device itself. They are subtle, about the size of a lipstick tube, and can be pulled out of a pocket at any time ready for use. I love these for impromptu magick, such as personal energy shielding. Their portability also makes them great for feeding spells from a distance.

Passive Diffusers

Passive diffusers are simply items from which essential oil can naturally disperse without any assistance. These include lava rocks, potpourri, felted wool balls, and reed diffusers. Passive diffusion is often overlooked because of its simplicity, but for a creative and magickal mind, the options for what can be used as a passive diffuser are almost endless. They are lovely when a more subdued type of supportive energy is needed. There is an ease and accessibility to them that infuses essential oils with gentle encouragement.

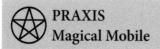 **PRAXIS
Magical Mobile**

Here is a magickal way to make a hanging mobile as a form of passive diffusion. The intention of this spell is to set a foundation from which all your work with aromatherapy will be built on: Learning from the wisdom of the past, listening to the lessons of the present, and leaning into the future with hope.

You'll need

- 3 lengths of ribbon, each about 12 inches long: one white to represent and honor ancestors, one green to represent oneself and a life of health and abundance, one black to represent and protect future descendants

- 3 drops of an essential oil you associate with ancestral connections. I recommend patchouli, vetiver, or rosemary

- 3 drops of an essential oil you associate with health and abundance. I recommend eucalyptus, peppermint, or lavender

- 3 drops of an essential oil you associate with vitality, inspiration, and protection. I recommend cinnamon, lemon, or melissa

- A stick or twig about 6 to 12 inches long with a string or fishing line tied to it for hanging

Directions

1. Hold the white ribbon and connect with your ancestors. Thank them for their support and wisdom. Send them your respect and honor them by dropping 3 drops of the ancestor's essential oil onto the ribbon. Tie it to the left side of the stick, knowing that they are supporting you.

2. Hold the green ribbon and connect to yourself, your body, your life in this moment. Send yourself some praise, and honor yourself by dropping 3 drops of the health and abundance essential oil onto the ribbon. Tie it to the center of the stick with gratitude for all that you have and are.

3. Hold the black ribbon and connect to your descendants. These are the makers of the future. Send them some encouragement and honor them by dropping 3 drops of the vitality, inspiration, and protection essential oil onto the ribbon. Tie it to the right side of the stick with a commitment to set them up as best you can.

4. Hang your mobile in a place where you can see and smell it. It could be above a doorway, in your garden, or above your altar.

May the experience of your mobile support your aromatherapy and magick with wisdom of the past, lessons of the present, and inspiration of the future unknown. So be it!

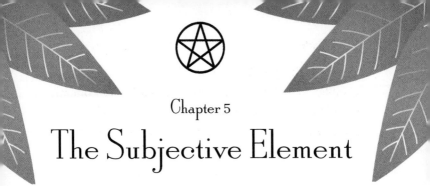

Chapter 5

The Subjective Element

Smell is often the first sense to inform us of something desirable nearby, and it also acts as the first line of defense against possible dangers. Before we are even aware that we are in contact with an aroma, the body has already received the input and has somehow reacted to it. Smell data is first taken into the nasal cavity and received by the only place in the human body where the central nervous system comes into direct contact with the outside environment, the olfactory epithelium. From there, smell signals are sent into the brain. Unlike other senses, smell signals go directly to the amygdala before being processed anywhere else. This part of the brain helps with decision making by managing memories and primal emotions like fear, sexual desire, anxiety, and aggression. Smell is a primordial sense. By gathering data with every breath taken in, it has helped us survive as a species. However, we are no longer in the primitive evolutionary stages of our existence.

As we have evolved, our minds have become more complex; our thoughts are more expansive and our emotions more nuanced. Our lives are much more complicated, and our experiences more diverse. These days, we all have a lot more internal clutter that we need to work through, process, and overcome. When we don't, that clutter can spill out into all areas of our lives and manifest in all kinds of unhelpful ways. By consciously using our sense of smell to resurface forgotten memories, to support emotional expression, to access trauma and deep reflexive responses, modern aromatherapy can help us address our individual and unique needs.

Experiencing Aroma

The effectiveness of aromatherapy relies heavily on the subjective element—our personal relationships with essential oils. As multi-faceted individuals, we have many aspects of self to take into consideration when using aromatherapy, especially when it's woven into a magickal practice. On top of that, there are several plant varieties available as essential oils that are all as complex as we are. Making blending choices can be a little intimidating. As mentioned in chapter 3, working with a professional spiritual aromatherapist makes this entire process much easier, since they already have the knowledge to guide you and the skill to objectively observe your responses and help you make sense of them. I'm going to walk you through my process and am confident that you will be able to adapt and implement it on your own with great success.

Before the oils even come out, I have my client fill out a standard health intake form addressing their current health status including acute issues, preexisting conditions, and health history. Then we talk about their spiritual path, belief system, practice, and any goals they may have. This discussion helps me narrow the field of essential oil options and lets me curate a selection for them to experience and assess through the lens of their subjective element.

The number of oils a client and I go through in a session is determined by the client's threshold for olfactory exhaustion. I might start with around five and add oils from there. It's important to allow some space and time to process the aromas and introspect a bit before moving on to the next. With each oil, we go through their physiological, psychological, emotional, spiritual, and magickal responses. I take a few minutes to ask prompting questions to help the client check in with their body and reflect on their experience. The more intense the responses, the fewer oils we evaluate in that session. Between each essential oil experience, we get fresh air and smell fresh coffee beans, which act as a palate cleanser.

When smelling an essential oil, don't stick your nose in it and sniff. Start by opening the bottle and wafting the aroma to your nose. You can even take in the scent from the bottle cap if you prefer, paying attention to how your mind, body, and spirit respond with each wafted inhalation.

The following is the order of elimination I use to narrow down scope of essential oils based on a person's subjective element:

Physiological Aspects
This category refers to the different ways in which bodies function—organs, muscles, hormones, health conditions, and so on. Questions might include "Does this aroma resonate anywhere in your physical body?" "Does it make you feel any colder or warmer?" "Can you intuit if there are any parts of your body that want more of this oil?"

Psychological Aspects
This category refers to the reactions in the mind that aromas can trigger. Smell memories, trauma from past experiences, likes and dislikes, et cetera. Questions for prompts might include "What is your first impression of this oil?" "Do any mental pictures come to mind when you smell it?" "What does it remind you of?"

Emotional Aspects

This item refers to mood and the way aromas make us feel: grounded, open to change, happy, and so on. Prompts might include "Has this aroma changed your emotional state in this moment?" "What is the dominant emotion it evokes?" "Can you connect that emotion to a reason why you might be feeling it?"

Aspects of Spirituality

This category refers to ways aromas are connected to our belief systems—historical uses, divine correlations, energy vibrations, et cetera. Exploring this aspect is when I rely most on my knowledge of how essential oils have been used spiritually in the past and why. Questions might include "Does this oil invoke any deity in particular?" "Can you sense any forms of energy around it?"

Aspects of Magickal Practice

This item refers to acts of worship or spiritual expression into which we can incorporate aromas: meditation, spellcraft, creation of sacred space, and more. This stage is when I most strongly rely on my experience as a Witch and Pagan minister. Prompt questions might include "Does this aroma resonate with a spiritual practice you already have?" "Do you have any practices that could be enhanced by this? If so, why?"

◆• •◆• •◆•

This order of operation nearly always works well. It starts with a plethora of essential oil options as we take into consideration the more general aspects of self. Then, as the aspects of self become more and more nuanced, the options narrow down.

Experiencing Aromas Demonstration: Melissa Officinalis

Following is an example of how the previous steps work in practice. I will be acting as my own client. Let's say I want to learn about how my subjective element responds to the essential oils of melissa (*Melissa officinalis*).

Step 1

Research potential risks and negative physiological interactions. Double check the client's health intake and cross reference with the contraindications of these essential oils. Assess any physical sensations or reactions that occur when experiencing the essential oil.

> *Known safety concerns for melissa:* Possible drug interaction and harmful to fetal health. Am I on medication or pregnant? No. I'll keep it as an option.

> *Physical sensations:* It makes my mouth water. I'll keep it.

Step 2 and Step 3

Our psychological impressions of an aroma are often linked to our emotions, so these can be evaluated together. Just make sure to make note of them separately. When evaluating oils for my own use, I find it helpful to speak my experience aloud in the moment as I'm experiencing it and make an audio recording.

> *Psychological impression:* Enjoyable aroma, smells juicy and makes me think of drinking herbal tea with friends. Gives a feeling of summer. Lemony, herbaceous, sweet. Keep as an option.
>
> *Emotional impression:* Makes me feel excited and motivated, like I want to go and experience something new. Keep as an option.

Step 4

This step involves documenting any spiritual correlations we may have learned or adopted from outside sources, such as historical or cultural associations. It also involves taking note of any intuitive correlations that arise while the client is smelling the oil. Make note of them separately.

> *Learned spiritual correlations:* Honey, bees, divination, Oracle of Delphi (ancient Greece)
>
> *Intuitive spiritual correlations:* Fae folk, jubilation, the time of year between Beltane and Midsummer

Step 5

Naturally, the next step is to discover where this oil might fit in well with the client's spiritual practices and magick. Often this is the point where a lot of inspiration pours in new ideas that could be integrated into current practices or used in the future. As your relationship with the essential oils deepen, much more will be revealed to you.

> *Magickal connection:* I had a strong connection and clear dialogue with this oil. It made me think of drinking herbal tea with friends. I felt a bit adventurous and motivated to experience something new. There is a link between melissa, bees, and divination.
>
> *Magickal practice:* It could be great for creating a sacred space for tasseomancy.

Experiencing Aromas Demonstration: Six Oils

What might this look like with other oils? Let's look at these five steps again using multiple oils including essential oils of grapefruit (*Citrus paradisii*), myrtle (*Myrtus communis*), juniper (*Juniperus communis*), sweet marjoram (*Origanum majorana*), ravintsara (*Cinnamomum camphora*), and nutmeg (*Myristica fragrans*).

Step 1

Consider the potential safety risks and physiological interactions.

Grapefruit

Safety considerations: Phototoxic if cold-expressed. Can I control where this will be applied to avoid skin that will be exposed to the sun? Yes. I'll keep it as an option.

Physical sensations: It makes my mouth water. I'll keep it.

Myrtle

Safety considerations: Some risk of toxicity accumulation. Do I want to preserve my liver and kidneys for metabolizing other things (like mead)? Yes.

Physical sensations: I'll remove this option without even smelling it.

Juniper

Safety considerations: Nothing significant physiologically to consider. I'll keep it.

Physical sensations: It's a bit nauseating. Nope, I'll take this option out.

Sweet Marjoram

Safety considerations: Nothing significant physiologically to consider. I'll keep it.

Physical sensations: I sense that it would feel good to rub it on my neck muscles. I'll keep it.

Ravintsara

Safety considerations: Can cause breathing difficulty and issues with the central nervous system of young children. Am I an adult? Yes. I'll keep it.

Physical sensations: My lungs love this! It stays.

Nutmeg

Safety considerations: In high doses, it can be psychotropic. At this point, if I knew we were not going to create a diffuser blend, bath oil or scrub, body lotion, or a similar method of use, I would keep this option. However, our magickal method of use has not been determined.

Physical sensations: I will remove it without even smelling it; I always err on the side of caution.

Step 2 and 3

In step 1, we eliminated myrtle, juniper, and nutmeg from our options. Now let's continue with the remaining oils. Here are some examples of reactions to the experience of these oils.

Grapefruit

Psychological impression: Smells like my mom's breakfast when I was a child. I remember her eating grapefruit halves with a weird serrated spoon.

A fond memory of my childhood home and family. Keep it.

Emotional impression: Makes me feel childlike, playful, and a little bit mischievous. Keep it.

Sweet Marjoram

Psychological impression: Enjoyable, herbaceous, sweet aroma. It makes me think of herbal sleeping pillows and getting ready for bedtime. Not cozy and cuddly vibes; more washing face and brushing teeth kind of vibes. I'll keep it.

Emotional impression: I feel calm and relaxed but also a bit task oriented. I feel like I am preparing for something. Keep it.

Ravintsara

Psychological impression: Full-on VapoRub and menthol cold lozenges experience. Fresh and stimulating aroma. Makes me think of fall and winter. Keep it.

Emotional impression: Makes me feel like I do when I have a cold, like I am emotionally trudging through, even though I just want to rest. Even though the psychological impression evoked a positive response, the emotional impression did not. I'll take this one out because I don't want to risk contaminating my magick with oils that prompted a negative reaction.

Step 4

In the last step, we eliminated ravintsara. Here are some examples of reactions to the experience of the two remaining oils:

Grapefruit

Learned spiritual correlations: None that I recall.

Intuitive spiritual correlations: Nothing comes to me.

Sweet Marjoram

Learned spiritual correlations: Joyous afterlife (ancient Greece)

Intuitive spiritual correlations: The liminal, easing transitions, Hekate (Greek mythology)

Step 5

Two oils remain. We will look at the potential magickal uses.

Grapefruit

Magickal connection: I'm not strongly connected to this oil; no profound communication. The fondness of my childhood home evokes childlike, playful, and mischievous energy.

Magickal practice: It could be good for shadow work that involves my inner child.

Sweet Marjoram

Magickal connection: A good connection, quiet but clear dialogue with this oil. It evoked a sense of preparing for rest. It made me feel calm and relaxed. It is associated with a joyous afterlife, the easing of transitions, and the goddess Hekate.

Magickal practice: This would be wonderful for death rites. Naturally, this includes helping our beloved dead cross over into the afterlife, but also for other deaths such as divorce, leaving a career, et cetera.

The more you work with your subjective element, the more you will notice that it is dynamic. Preferences change, new smell memories are made, and the way scent associations are processed shifts. Our relationships with aroma evolve over time. It is important to do a little check-in and reassess our subjective element every time we use aromatherapy, magickal or not.

Subjective Pentacle Blending Experiments

When I teach workshops, I like to break students into small groups to do experience experiments that highlight the subjective element of aromatherapy. Every table gets a selection of essential oils in numbered bottles along with a worksheet that has corresponding numbered columns. We start by choosing one oil that everybody will smell. Without discussion, we jot down our initial thoughts and individual impressions, including things that will help us learn about our subjective element, such as linked memories. Is the aroma pleasing or is it unenjoyable? What vibes does it give off? Are there any intuitive messages that come through?

We repeat this process for each numbered oil. After we've worked through each one, we compare our worksheets to see how similarly (and differently) we perceived and responded to the same aromas. It's an incredible experiment! It bonds us as a group and highlights our individual uniqueness.

For the next level of this group experiment, we take what we've learned about our subjective elements to create pentacle blends. Independently, everyone decides how they might arrange the oils as they relate to the pentacle using one of the following correlation sets.

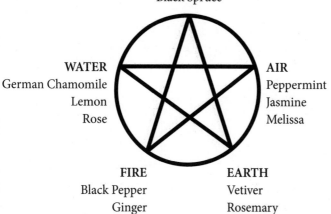

SPIRIT
Frankincense
Sandalwood
Black Spruce

WATER
German Chamomile
Lemon
Rose

AIR
Peppermint
Jasmine
Melissa

FIRE
Black Pepper
Ginger
Pine

EARTH
Vetiver
Rosemary
Patchouli

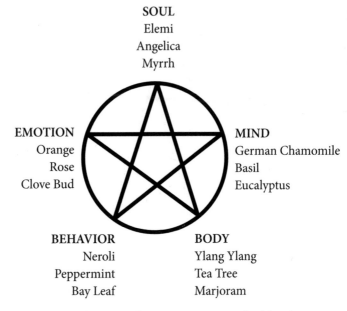

SOUL
Elemi
Angelica
Myrrh

EMOTION
Orange
Rose
Clove Bud

MIND
German Chamomile
Basil
Eucalyptus

BEHAVIOR
Neroli
Peppermint
Bay Leaf

BODY
Ylang Ylang
Tea Tree
Marjoram

Once we've each created a custom pentacle blend on paper, we share and compare our answers and discuss our individual processes of reasoning: "Why did you choose to put black pepper in the earth element?" "Why did you choose to put black pepper in the fire element?" It is a fun introduction to how differently we experience essential oils and brings attention to the importance of the subjective element. What we do with these discoveries depends on the group. If the individuals in the group are a collective, like a coven or a family, we might co-create a blend that represents their collective. They would then be able to use it in whatever future magickal workings they wanted.

If the group is made of strangers, folks might decide to use the pentacle data to blend something magickal for themselves. What I like most about using a pentacle to essential oil blending is that it will reveal possibilities that we might not think of on our own. I first discovered one of my favorite essential oil combos, rose and lime, this way. I invite you to try this experiment with friends. As you continue working through the book, you'll see it the foundation of my approach to aromatherapy and magick.

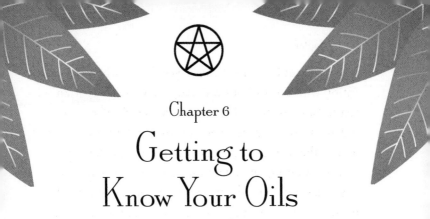

Chapter 6

Getting to Know Your Oils

As your relationship with essential oils strengthens, it becomes easier to ask them questions and get an accurate understanding of what they can offer in terms of support and guidance. We should all strive to improve communication between ourselves and the oils so that clear messages are transferred between us.

When we are working with magick, it is important that the oils be made aware of our intentions. Remember, these are little plant souls waiting for instructions. We need to inform them what we are doing and hope they will offer support. In other words, we need their consent to respectfully work with them.

My technique for getting consent is to pick up the oil, put it in the palms of my prayer hands, take it up to my third eye, inform it of my goals and intentions, and ask if it would be willing to contribute to the magick. If the oil's response is no, I say thank you for clearly communicating with me and put it down. I have also experienced referrals, when an oil has recommended a different oil for the job as well as times when the oils told me exactly how to use them to get optimal results. Again, the stronger your relationship with your oils, the easier it is to get clear answers from them. If you aren't confident in interpreting the oils' consent messages, using a pendulum can be helpful to get confirmation. Before using, establish how the pendulum will communicate yes and no, then hold it over each oil and ask the pendulum if the oil gives consent to be used in whatever way you are hoping to use it.

Building Friendships

Getting to know your oils is one of the most rewarding parts of building a magickal aromatherapeutic practice. This is not about knowing what's in your cupboard, what's on the bottle labels, or even what the oil's medicinal properties are. Getting to know your oils is about relationship building. As spiritual practitioners, it's not unusual to communicate with non-living things psychically, empathically, and intuitively. We do this with all our magickal tools to some degree—our tarot cards, crystals, and ritual knives, for example. None of these things are technically living, but we can feel their energy and interact with them to develop powerful bonds. With time, we can get to know our oils with the same kind of magickal dialogue.

When we first meet a new person, we usually don't spend hours and hours getting to know each other and dive into the depths of who we are. Relationship building takes time and space because we need to be able to process our thoughts and feelings in the context of our new friendship. When getting to know essential oils, I find that spending several relatively short periods of time together is much more manageable. This approach nurtures our developing bond, instead of forcing it.

It is much easier to get to know an essential oil than it is to get to know another person. Humans are complex and complicated beings. Essential oils are also complex, but they are not complicated or judgmental. They are always direct and are only motivated by their inherent purpose, to heal. Although essential oils are straightforward friends, our relationships with them are still dynamic.

Expect that your relationship with them will sometimes change, although always remaining impactful. I still remember my first encounters with a blend from my first aromatherapy job twenty-five-ish years ago. I absolutely hated that blend. How much I hated it was so obvious that my boss interceded and suggested that I get to know it a little better and show it a little kindness. I was dubious. This was before I had integrated aromatherapy into my magickal practices, but as a Witch I was open to seemingly bizarre suggestions like that. So, I took their advice and started to greet that shitty blend every day.

When I arrived at work, I'd have a brief conversational interaction with it, and then carry on with my day. It looked something like "Hello Blendy McBlenderson, how are you today? I hope it is going to be a great one for you. So far, my day is OK. I am feeling a little tired, but generally happy and healthy … alrighty then … I guess I'll smell ya later!" I would literally speak to it, out loud, and send it a little respect and gratitude. Sometimes, I would pick it up and experience its aroma and, instead of reacting in a visibly negative way, I would consciously send it a little more love and appreciation for all its healing gifts.

After some time, I started to pick up some energetic responses from it. I was receiving impressions that were helping me understand it better. I felt an empathy and connection to it that was growing. It was becoming clear that our relationship was improving because I no longer hated the blend's aroma. I even started to enjoy it! I spent more time with it and our relationship grew stronger, so I started using it in my life outside of work. Not long after, it became my favorite blend. The progression of my relationship with that essential oil blend is still impactful and before my boss made that suggestion, I never even considered my interpersonal relationships with oils. Even though the advice I received wasn't expected to resonate the way that it did, it was wise and magickal. Looking back, I wish I had journaled the experience.

Techniques for Relationship Building

I am going to share some techniques for essential oil relationship building. I invite you to use some kind of journal as you are getting to know your oils. Especially considering how helpful it is to have a historical record of your essential oil impressions when learning about your subjective element. Know that the following techniques don't need to be done in the order that they're written. They aren't dependent on each other, but naturally, I recommend that you try them all because I want you to have the ultimate essential oil bonding experience. If you aren't going to try them all, consider trying at least a few different techniques to connect and communicate with your oils. Each approach will yield different results.

Initial Investigation

One way to start getting a better understanding of essential oils is to learn about the plant species from which they are extracted. This is a great place to start since you don't even need any oils to do it, you just need to have the name of an oil that you're interested in. All that this initial investigation involves is a little research. What does the essential oil plant source look like? How does it grow? How does it propagate? Which environmental conditions does it grow best in? What part(s) of the plant are distilled to extract essential oil? What insects does it attract or repel? Jot down what you learn in your grimoire.

Here's an example of what the grimoire entry might look like for vetiver essential oil.

Vetiveria zizanioides
- is a grass, evergreen, perennial herb, looks a bit like lemongrass.
- grows in clumps up to 5 ft high and wide.
- essential oil distilled from roots.
- roots are long, fine, and very strong.
- roots grow down 13 ft and can sometimes do it in their first year.
- plants are tough! Can withstand flood and drought conditions, frosts and wildfires, and heavy animal grazing.
- roots loosen compacted soil while preventing erosion.
- can help rehabilitate metal-polluted and fuel-polluted soil.

Next, look over your findings and jot down some intuitive, but logical, assumptions about what might be some of the essential oil's energetic properties. When I look at the above list of traits for vetiver, I would expect that it is extremely grounding and would make one feel safe. I think it could offer a resilient kind of strength that would help one endure challenging times. It may have a rehabilitating healing aspect that would be helpful to folks in recovery from substance abuse.

Continuing the investigation, consider its history and culture. Where is it from? When has it been used and by whom? How has it been used in the past? After you've collected a good amount of intriguing data, reread it once more to see if anything specific stands out. Perhaps you'll see striking parallels to your initial intuitive hunches, or perhaps your first impressions will transform in the light of newfound details. At this point, the mystery surrounding the essential oils you've researched starts to fade. I'd venture to say that you're now on familiar terms with them.

Interviewing

To deepen this acquaintance, your next step would be to take in the aromas. There are two parts to this technique, both of which require a smell experience of the essential oils. The first part is learning about your subjective element, which chapter 5 covered in detail. If you haven't already started to explore and journal your subjective element, this is the time to do it.

When smelling an essential oil, remember to waft the aroma to your nose. Paying attention to your mind, body, and spirit with each inhale, record any physical responses, psychological and emotional reactions, spiritual impressions, and magickal associations. Make sure to also jot down a brief aromatic description of the oil. An aromatic description for vetiver might be smoky, deep, sweet notes, slightly floral, and reminiscent of charcoal.

The second part of this technique involves directly communicating with the oil. We want to learn about motivation and purpose from the perspective of the oil. Holding the open bottle in your hands, ask the oil a few questions that will help you understand how it wants to heal and what impacts it wants to make. Active questions seek to know what to do about something, while passive questions seek to learn about the way something is or will be. I like to ask both kinds and, of course, record the results in my grimoire. For example, my communication with vetiver could look like this:

I hold the bottle between my palms with my hands in a prayer position. I ground myself, get centered, and bring my hands up to my forehead over my third eye. With the bottle in my palms and the back of my thumbs touching my forehead, I speak to the oil; in this case, vetiver:

> *Passive Question:* What is your healing purpose?
>
> *Vetiver's Answer:* Equal energy moving up and down, balancing the celestial and terrestrial to find a spiritual center, connecting the mind to body and body to mind, evoking safety and lowered anxiety.
>
> *Active Question:* What can I do to help you achieve your healing purpose?

Vetiver's Answer: When a person is experiencing something extreme, it can feel precarious and unsafe. I work best as a counterbalance, a solid anchor point on the opposing side of chaos. This will help one feel safer and give them courage in the face of something that feels out of control and dangerous.

My Response: Thank you for all your awesomeness and for communicating with me. I am really looking forward to growing our relationship further.

Now that I've learned these things about my vetiver essential oil, its qualities will more easily come to mind when I'm in need of its unique ways of healing. When I look back in my grimoire to the results of the vetiver investigation, I see that this communication aligns with my initial impressions. It would work well to support folks through challenging times, a particularly caring companion when moving through grief. Seeking a deeper understanding of an essential oil's divine purpose helps us tap into their inherent healing magick, which in turn adds power to our own.

Sharing Stories

As we deepen our human connections with one another, trust gradually emerges and grows. We start new relationships with casual exchanges that demand little trust from either party until eventually we reach a point where we feel secure enough to reveal our soft underbellies. A similar progression takes place in the realm of essential oils but without any apprehension linked to vulnerability. The only requisite is to be receptive to your essential oils and narrate a few chapters from your life's story.

For me to differentiate my voice more clearly from the essential oil's voice, I find it much easier to share my stories out loud. Keep in mind that while we communicate our thoughts and experiences with words, the essential oils may communicate their stories in a different way. Sharing stories is reciprocal—take the time to listen. One great way to listen is journey work.

Journeying

This ancient and global practice lets us interact with spirits, guides, and other divine forms. It can involve deep meditation, visualization, and often trancelike states. To help us listen to our essential oils, I recommend the following technique, which is based on the sacred practice of journeying. Although it's not required, it can be helpful to have an experienced spiritual aromatherapist with you, to act as a guide and anchor.

The process begins with setting the intention, defining what you hope to achieve through the journey. This is an important step in order to receive clear communication from the essential oil. Once you've set your intention, it's time to find an oil that wants to join you on the journey. There are different ways to do this: you could ask your spiritual aromatherapist to recommend an oil, or you could take an intuitive approach and allow yourself to be guided by your instincts.

Once you've identified the oil that is ready to share in this experience, it's time to physically prepare for the journey. First, you'll want to create a sacred space where you can relax and be free of distractions. It may seem contrary, but I find it much easier to listen to an essential oil if I am inside while journeying, not outside in nature. Place a few items in the sacred space that will assist you in your journey, such as a diffuser, an audio recorder, your journaling grimoire, and a pencil, maybe even a sketch pad for drawing. I prefer to actively diffuse in a nebulizer when journeying because it fills the space with an undiluted vapor of my selected essential oil. Once the space is set and the oil of the journey is filling the air, you're ready to begin.

Sitting up or laying down, get comfortable, close your eyes, and allow yourself to drift into a light trancelike state. Take deep breaths and focus on the intention set at the beginning of this process. Visualize the spirit of the essential oil and let it know that you are there to listen. Psychically open yourself up to any messages, images, or sensations that come through. For now, just observe and listen to the communications instead of getting involved in a dialogue. Allow the visions to flow freely through your consciousness—there is no need to hold on to any of it. It is possible that you will find yourself sharing your stories with the oil at this time, too. However, journeying is a skill. I suggest just listening during your first essential oil journey. Build some trust and understanding about what that experience looks like for you before trying to share and listen in the same session. When the story sharing feels complete, you can end the journey by thanking the oil spirit for journeying with you and return to your awareness to your physical body. Ground yourself. Reflect on what you experienced and write down any insights. A lot of magickal memory can be lost in just a couple of minutes and you'll need quality notes that you can review and use later.

The ways in which the oils communicate on the meditative journey will continue to develop for a while after the experience. Processing the journey is an important part and is how we make sense of it in the context of our lives. A week or so after the journey, I recommend meditating lightly on the experience. This meditation is not another journey; it doesn't need to go deep. We just want to quiet the mind enough to allow anything from the journey that's floating around in our subconscious to surface. The insights, reflections, resolutions, and deep understanding that can emerge in us after journeying with essential oils can be profound. In my perception, venturing with the spirits of essential oils feels strikingly different from journeying with the spirits of living or harvested whole plants. Facilitated by this practice, you and your oils will develop whole new levels of mutual awareness and connection.

Those Who Divine Together, Align Together

Aromatherapy and divination games make for an unconventional bonding exercise. They broaden the spectrum of how we engage with our oils, enriching our relationships with them. These games also serve as an efficient tool for refining our intuitive instincts and psychic abilities. I suggest jotting down the outcomes as well to keep track of your progress.

For many, the practice of divination is quite reverent. We are focused, centered, and tapped into the source. What I like about this method of essential oil relationship building is that I get to play with my essential oils and divination tools in a very casual way. It's refreshing and fun. The divination tools that I find most effective for this are tarot or oracle cards and pendulums.

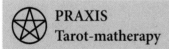 **PRAXIS**
Tarot-matherapy

I call this aromatherapy divination game "Tarot-matherapy." It's played by setting out a variety of essential oils and asking your cards to make a match between the predominant qualities of the essential oils and the predominant interpretations of the tarot cards. The intention is to discover conceptual analogies and harmonious pairings of oils and cards through divination. I have never done this with anyone who didn't already have a deck of tarot cards that they regularly use. In theory, that shouldn't matter as long as you know how to use and interpret the tarot you are using.

You'll need

- 3 distinctly different essential oils
- A deck of tarot cards
- 3 index cards or blank paper and a pen
- Your grimoire

Directions

1. Gameplay starts with the oil setup. Smell an oil, connect to it, inform it of the game's intention, and establish the three most dominant qualities that you are going to assign to it.

2. Jot those qualities down on an index card and set the oil bottle on it so that you don't have to remember those qualities while playing. Repeat this and the previous step for each of the remaining essential oils.

3. Ground and center, then pick up your tarot deck. Connect with the cards just as you would if you were about to do a reading. Inform them of the game's intention and start to shuffle. You can do this with all the cards, or just the major arcana.

4. Ask the cards to provide you with a good match for one of the oils, pull the card but don't look at it yet—place it face down with the oil.

5. Do this for all the oils until each one has three cards.

6. Then, grab your grimoire to record the results and flip over the cards. Which matches immediately make sense? Don't worry if the matches aren't immediately powerful. The primary purpose of this exercise is to build the relationships between you, your oils, and your cards. The secondary purpose is to receive helpful information and guidance.

Tarot-matherapy Example

Here are the three oils that I chose along with the three qualities that I most strongly associate with them:

Sweet orange oil: Big sun energy, joyous, playfulness
Eucalyptus oil: Refresh, awaken, vitality
Patchouli oil: Times past, roots, growth

Next, I pulled three cards for each of those essential oils. As I flipped the cards over to reveal them, I noticed how *most* of them felt like a perfect pair and it was obvious why they were matched.

Sweet orange oil: Four of Rods, the Chariot, Eight of Swords

Eucalyptus oil: The Fool, Two of Swords, Knight of Rods

Patchouli oil: Two of Rods, King of Cups, Four of Swords

During the initial round of card-drawing, the Eight of Swords surfaced as a match for orange oil and in the subsequent round, the Two of Swords emerged for the eucalyptus oil. These did not immediately make sense to me. In the deck I was using, the Eight of Swords shows a woman bound and blindfolded. There is water pooled at her feet, and she is surrounded by eight swords forming a barrier around her. This does not reflect the joyous, playful, sun energy that I attribute to sweet orange essential oil. This presented an opportunity to do some introspection. I needed to examine the card more intimately through my subjective lens and in the context of my life.

Looking inward, I asked questions such as: What is going on with me that might be calling out for the orange oil's healing? Is the orange oil reaching out to say "Hey, I can help you with this"? Here I interpret the Eight of Swords card as a symbol of self-imposed mental barriers. As I ponder the connection between it and the orange oil through the lens of my current life experiences, it becomes clear: the card is mirroring my own struggles with self-doubt and insecurity while writing this book. The orange oil recognizes my need for healing, to dissolve my mental blocks and to embrace the joy in self-expression.

I interpret the Two of Swords card as a message of uncertainty with the need for contemplation, often because an informed decision needs to be made. This makes complete sense in the context of my current situation. The eucalyptus oil reminds me that it will help clear any mental clutter and bring the clarity I need.

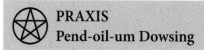

PRAXIS
Pend-oil-um Dowsing

I call this next aromatherapy divination game Pend-oil-um Dowsing. It can help you calibrate or align with your pendulum, tune in to the energies of essential oils, and expand your psychic abilities. The game's objective is to identify the standout essential oil through divination.

You'll need

- 3 essential oils with similar aromatic profiles and healing qualities
- 1 essential oil in stark contrast to the other three (example: 3 citrus oils, plus patchouli)
- A pendulum
- Your grimoire

Directions

1. Smell an oil, connect to it, inform it of the game's intention and establish one quality that you are going to assign to it and the other three similar oils. (Example: fresh, invigorating, or light.)

2. Then smell the standout oil, connect to it, inform it of the game's intention and establish one *contrasting* quality that you are going to assign. (Example: earthy, grounding, or sedative.)

3. Keep the bottle labels visible and place them in a row about 6 inches apart. Then run your magickal hand(s) over the oils, pausing over each one to state the name and quality while sensing its vibrations.

4. Calibrate your pendulum to respond "no" to the similar oils and "yes" to the standout oil. Establish its neutral starting position and ask for it to show the movement for "yes." Then, have it show the "no" movement.

5. Next, pick up the standout oil and hold it with the pendulum in the palms of your hands. Communicate to the pendulum that this oil should elicit a "yes" response, then test it. Go through this calibration process with each of the remaining oils, informing the pendulum

that they should elicit "no" responses. Proceed to the next step when you feel confident that you, the oils, and the pendulum are all in complete understanding of the task.

6. Cover the oil bottles with a little piece of cloth or a tissue and move them around, shuffling their position in the lineup. Even better, have someone else do this for you while you are not in the room.

7. Run your magickal hand(s) over the bottles and jot down what you sense. Then ground, center, and connect with your pendulum reminding it of its divinatory purpose. Use it to locate the standout oil, writing about its responses in your grimoire. Before you unveil the oil bottles, check to see if what your magickal hands picked as the standout oil is the same as what the pendulum says. Then uncover the bottles to check your accuracy.

As you continue to practice divination and aromatherapy, your understanding of the oils will deepen, and the stronger your psychic and dowsing abilities will become.

Options Overload

One possible problem with getting to know essential oils is that you might want *all* of them. Just remember that in aromatherapy, the quality of the essential oils is much more important than quantity, and this is especially true when we use them for magick. It's rare, but if they aren't treated with respect, it's possible they could take on some vibes of neglect and that negative energy might contaminate your good works. Each individual essential oil has many healing properties, and it is very possible to find a single high-quality oil that will work for a wide array of magickal options.

My advice is to first use your intuition and ask yourself, "if I could only have one essential oil, what would it be and why?" It is possible that oil is the one that will best serve you across a wide spectrum of magickal needs. Alternatively, try the following technique to isolate the one oil to rule them all. Here are some techniques for finding "the One Oil," also referred to as "my preciouussssss."

Review Your Practice

Jot down the three to five spiritual practices that you do most often in a month. If you do several different acts of magick monthly, you might be looking at your calendar thinking "how do I narrow all this down to a top five?!" In this context, if the magickal acts/spiritual practices have the same general intention, they count as one. When categorized by intention, very few people regularly do more than five different acts of magick each month.

For instance, if every month I did a short daily meditation, a full moon rite, and a form of magick for cleansing/

protecting my home, I would count three magickal acts. If a busy medium does twenty readings each month, daily devotions at their ancestor altar, plus a cleansing/protecting ritual every week, the total count is also three magickal acts, not fifty-four. Again, magickal acts/spiritual practices with the same general intention count as one.

Review Your Intentions

Once you have defined the number of monthly acts/practices, write the intention of each as a column heading. You might have just one column, and that is fine. Up to five is enough for this exercise. Using my previous example, I would make three column headings: Cleansing and Protecting Spell, Full Moon Rite, and Daily Devotions.

Next, break down each practice into smaller parts, the factors that contribute to the success of each intention. I consider this a form of shadow work. For example, under the column titled "Cleansing/Protecting Spell," I would list a breakdown of its smaller goals:

- Dispel negativity and fear
- Detach unfriendly attachments
- Shield from the ill-natured
- Invite positivity and joy
- Fortify strength
- Encourage bravery
- Foster love

- Bring peace
- Feel safe

Match Your Goals to Oils

Next, examine the list of goals and think about what essential oil might work well to address them. It's probable that a couple of different oils will come to mind. As an experienced aromatherapist, when I subjectively look at my sample list of smaller goals, I know that rose essential oil would serve well to address all those things. Other options might be juniper, rosemary, and frankincense. Performing these analyses is where your knowledge of essential oil properties and your personal relationships with them will really make a difference.

Let's walk through the last steps again using another one of my column headings, "Full Moon Rite." I would break it down into a list of its smaller goals. The goals within my Full Moon Rite column are:

- Connect with the Divine within and around me
- Express gratitude for my emotions
- Heal emotional hurts and trauma
- Connect with the ocean
- Feel grounded
- Embrace my personal power
- Celebrate Nature's beauty

Next, I examine the above list and choose some essential oils that would help me achieve those ritual goals. Because I am trying to identify one multi-tasking oil, I start by checking if rose oil might work well for any of these, too. Notice that it would indeed work wonderfully, yay! Frankincense, neroli, and sandalwood would also be great options.

One last time, let's go through the steps together starting at my next column with the heading "Daily Devotions." I would break down my intentions into a list of goals:

- Get centered
- Connect with my true purpose
- Send love to my ancestors and other guides
- Feel and express gratitude
- Commune with the five elements of Nature

I once again examine these goals and identify what essential oils would be a good match (step 4). Would rose oil work for these? For the most part, I say yes. I don't necessarily think that rose oil would help me commune with the elements of nature, but it certainly wouldn't hurt. Sandalwood, frankincense, and patchouli would be lovely, too.

Looking at all my options, I then look for the most crossover. Rose oil stands out as "my preciousssss" and would be my first pick. However, rose essential oil is quite expensive, and if I only have a small collection of oils, I will probably use a lot of it. No probbies! Frankincense is just as perfect a choice to be my One Oil.

As you start this, it may seem a little unlikely that you could discover a single essential oil to address most of the goals and intentions of your magickal work. The fact is that essential oils are extremely versatile and adaptable. Every one of them has overlapping properties that affect us and our magick on both the physical and metaphysical planes. The complex makeup of an essential oil allows us to use them in a variety of ways. We can use them in an expansive manner to benefit from their broad-reaching effects, or we can focus on more subtle aspects and uses to finely tune our practices. With the myriad options available for both witchcraft and aromatherapy, finding "the one oil to rule them all" is a great way to avoid overwhelm and just get started.

Chapter 7

Forms of Aromatherapy and Magick

I define magick as a spiritual act or occurrence. Magick can be active or passive, intentional or circumstantial. Sometimes the word "magick" could be used synonymously with "a special moment," "luck," or "blessing," and I have certainly experienced it in all those ways and more. When I am teaching about my approach to aromatherapy, I often use the words "magick" and "spiritual" interchangeably. I am not doing this because I think they are the same, but because I think that they originate from the same place inside us.

I believe that all people experience spirituality on a regular basis regardless of their belief systems. In fact, it could be that our belief systems are built around our spiritual experiences as a way for us to make sense of them. When something spiritual is happening, we feel it. It's that feeling of total awe that fills the chest and tingles on the skin and is sometimes so intense that it's almost too much to bear. It's an overwhelming sense that tells us that we are taking part in something truly special: the moment when we first catch sight of fireflies flickering in the twilight, stroke the incredible silkiness of a puppy's ear, tune in to the entrancing melody of a whale's song, or sink into the comforting warmth of a long-awaited embrace from a loved one. Wherever that irrefutable spiritual sensation is emanating from is the same source that gives birth to magick, and it's inextricably connected to pure, unbridled, and overflowing gratitude. As practitioners of the magickal arts, we engage with that vital energy. We endeavor to elevate, channel, and direct it to make positive change.

Most of my magickal practices fit into seven categories: energetic healing, meditation, rituals, rites, spellcraft, communing, shadow work, and divination. However, I can't think of a single magickal practice that wouldn't work wonderfully with an aromatherapeutic accompaniment. When we use essential oils in a magickal way, their energy and that of the practitioner, recipient, and the energy behind the intention all contribute to the power being raised. Because of this, the clear and focused visualization of our intention plays a major role.

Shadow Work

With all forms of magick, the clarity of intention and consistency of the spiritual work are critical. If our goals and actions aren't clear and aligned, the work won't be as successful. This is why I believe that shadow work can be an important contributing factor to magickal practice. It's important to understand our potentially hidden motivations, what aspects of ourselves are showing up and why. Only when we are nonjudgmentally honest about ourselves can we get truly clear on our intentions.

I often incorporate shadow work into my spiritual practices. It marries well with magick as they both seek to unveil and work with the mysteries of ourselves and the universe. Shadow work can be achieved through various methods, including journaling, meditation, dream work, energy work, breath work, and psychotherapy. Shadow work as a practice has been around for a long time, gaining popularity in recent years as more people are looking to explore their inner depths.

Shadow work involves exploring the parts of ourselves that we have denied or repressed out of fear so that we can reclaim and integrate them into our lives. It's an exploration that can be both empowering and challenging. When we take on shadow work, we can come to understand ourselves more deeply and gain clarity on our life paths. It is an opportunity to keep discovering and becoming more of who we truly are. I believe that when combined with spiritual practices, shadow work is one of the most powerful and transformative tools for self-discovery, healing, and growth. When incorporating shadow work into your life and spiritual practice, it is important to take care with yourself and not push too hard. Take your time and be gentle, approaching your shadows with curiosity instead of judgment. They are an integral part of who you are, and embracing them should bring a newfound sense of self-love, understanding, and acceptance.

Energetic Healing

Energetic healing is a holistic approach that centers on maintaining and restoring life force or vitality. It aims to bring balance to the numerous energy points, fields, and streams that contribute to our physical, emotional, and spiritual health. Forms of energy healing include acupuncture, acupressure, reiki, touch therapy, vibrational medicine, auric cleansing, and chakra balancing. These practices interact with the subtle energy aspects of humans, addressing energy system disruptions. Energetic healing suggests that when our life force is strong and flowing, we can better handle life's difficulties.

My method of aromatherapy and magick is rooted in the belief that the well-being of our energetic selves is as important as the health of the mind, emotions, and body. When the strength of our energy body is improved and our energy centers better aligned, we can attune more easily to other energy forms. Just like us, essential oils have their own inherent energy. They too can move energy, take it in, send it out, and transform it. The healing effects of essential oils complement energetic healing principles. Like concentrated forms of plant vitality, when used in energetic healing, essential oils can help balance the flow of energy across our systems. Their unique vibrations can interact with our energy field, initiating a healing process that reaches all aspects of our being. Here is an example of how I might choose essential oils to attune to the chakras.

Root Chakra

This is the first chakra, it can be visualized as the color red. It is located at the base of the spine and torso, the groin area. The root chakra is the closest to the earth and is connected to the sense of security, foundation, and physical needs. When choosing an essential oil that relates to this chakra, I might want one to help with grounding—patchouli, vetiver, or carrot seed.

Sacral Chakra

This is the second chakra and it can be visualized as the color orange. It is located just below the belly button. The sacral chakra is the emotional center and is connected to feelings, creativity, and desire. When choosing an essential oil that relates to this chakra, I might want one to encourage the expression of those things—clary sage, sweet orange, or ylang-ylang.

Solar Plexus Chakra

This is the third chakra and can be visualized as the color yellow. It is located at the solar plexus muscles just above the belly button. The solar plexus chakra is the center of personal power and is connected to self-esteem, motivation, and a sense of purpose. When choosing an essential oil that relates to this chakra, I might want one to help with empowerment—Australian sandalwood, black pepper, or ginger.

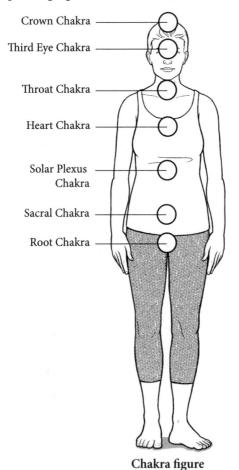

Crown Chakra

Third Eye Chakra

Throat Chakra

Heart Chakra

Solar Plexus Chakra

Sacral Chakra

Root Chakra

Chakra figure

Heart Chakra

This is the fourth chakra and can be visualized as the color green. It is located at the sternum in the chest. The heart chakra is the relationships center and is connected to love, empathy, and personal growth. When choosing an essential oil that relates to this chakra, I might want one to resonate deep healing—rose, rose, or rose (just kidding). Other good oils are palmarosa and jasmine.

Throat Chakra

This is the fifth chakra and can be visualized as the color blue. It is located at the throat, the vocal cord area. The throat chakra is the center of communication and is connected to expressing oneself, individual truth, and social skills. When choosing an essential oil that relates to this chakra, I might want one to help with composure—German chamomile, lavender, or geranium.

Third Eye Chakra

This is the sixth chakra and can be visualized as the color indigo, a bluish purple. It is located in the middle of the forehead. The third eye chakra is the center of foresight and is connected to intuition, decision making, and wisdom. When choosing an essential oil that relates to this chakra, I might want one to help with clarity—basil, helichrysum, or cypress.

Crown Chakra

This is the seventh chakra and can be visualized as the color violet. I see it as luminous and radiating with pure white light, the unification of all prismatic colors. It is located slightly above the top of the head, like a crown. The crown chakra is the nexus of the Divine within and around. It is the center of spiritual connectedness. The crown chakra is the closest to the cosmos and corresponds to the higher self, enlightenment, and serenity. So, when choosing an essential oil that relates to this chakra, I might want one to help with divine attunement—frankincense, angelica root, or bay leaf.

Meditation

This ancient and sacred practice is aimed at cultivating inner harmony and spiritual well-being. It awakens our senses, evokes tranquility, and draws us into a realm of profound peace. Now, imagine elevating this potent ritual by combining it with the magick of essential oils. Aromatherapy can remarkably intensify our meditative journeying, creating a sensory experience that transcends the ordinary. When deeply drawn through our nostrils, each inhalation of essential oils is invited to mingle with our internal universe. Their journey from the external world to the depths of our mind is a profound one. Motivated to heal, they make their way straight to our brain, the command center of our cognition and perception. They create a conducive environment within the brain, paving the way for meditation to do its restorative work. To achieve this, I think diffusion is the most effective method of aromatherapy to use with meditation. There are two key techniques for diffusion: passive and active.

As I shared in chapter 4, passive diffusion offers a gentle whisper of scents that allows essential oils to naturally evaporate, subtly infusing our surroundings. Active diffusion disperses essential oils into our environment in a dynamic aromatic cloud that quickly reaches every corner of a room. My meditation practices are usually either intended to clear the mind, self-heal, or manifest. The choice between passive and active diffusion depends on the rhythm of my meditation, like choosing between a soothing lullaby or an energetic melody. In a meditation to clear the mind, for instance, I could either invoke an active blustery air energy or a passive falling-leaves type of energy.

Here are some examples of how you might use the nature of the diffusion method to reinforce the intention of your meditations.

Meditating to Clear the Mind

This type of meditation requires a quiet space and the ability to acknowledge and let go of any thoughts or emotions. Using a bowl of warm water, passively diffuse an essential oil blend that helps you release your thoughts, surrender control, and help you feel grounded and secure. Patchouli and sweet marjoram might be lovely for this.

Sit in a cross-legged position and hold the bowl in your lap. Find the aromas in the air with your inhale, visualizing any unhelpful thoughts or emotions being encapsulated by the patchouli and marjoram (or whatever essential oils you choose). On exhale, release those thoughts or emotions, surrounded by the caring spirit of the essential oils. Visualize any voids in your energy body being filled with their quiet, calm, grounded energy.

Meditating to Self-Heal

This method requires focus and a sense of purpose. If you are working on healing anxiety, for example, you would want to actively diffuse a blend that would calm your nerves, help you focus, and connect to the Divine. Neroli and frankincense in a nebulizer could work well.

Lay down somewhere comfortable and set a timer for thirty minutes, or a shorter time period if you prefer. Begin by visualizing the neroli essence (or other essential oils) going into your brain and soothing your nervous system. Picture all of your overactive and frazzled nerve signals becoming smooth, controlled, and focused. As the neroli continues to ease any inner chaos, seek out the aroma of the frankincense. Visualize it as divine white light all around that assures you that *you are safe*. As it fills your entire being, remember that *you have choice*. Remain like that for the duration of the session, slowly and deliberately breathing, allowing the aromas to gently remind you that *everything will be just fine*.

Meditating to Manifest

Manifesting peace, in this example, requires controlled and clear visualizations. Choose a peacemaking blend to use in an ultrasonic diffuser. My blend includes essential oils of patchouli, myrrh, rose, and Roman chamomile.

Let the experience of the aromas guide your visualizations. Speak aloud "I feel the patchouli digging roots into the earth and grounding me. I feel the myrrh connecting me to the energy of the universe. I invite the rose to warm and open my heart as the chamomile calms my fears." Then use your focused thoughts to create peace by taking relevant examples of non-peace and transforming them in your mind. Visualize anger becoming compassion, weapons becoming flowers, and hitting becoming hugging. Allow yourself to feel differently about something that upsets you. Let your feelings of love, understanding, and genuine caring spread out over the world, seeing all people feeling safe and comfortable. Say this aloud, knowing it to be true: "I am manifesting peace in myself and all around me."

•✦• •✦• •✦•

As you can see with all these methods, the overall goal is to connect some specific healing aspects of the essential oils and the method of use to enhance the meditation objective. There are endless opportunities for synergy; the more we practice, the easier it becomes.

Rituals

Rituals serve as our anchors, connecting us to the world around us and offering solace in the predictability of their occurrence. Repeated practices such as daily devotions, weekly deity-day worship, monthly energy cleansing of the home, and lunar events, integrate our spiritual beliefs into the rhythm of our lives. Despite their repetition, every ritual is special and holds a powerful purpose with an opportunity for spiritual elevation. Essential oils add a fragrant experience to these recurring ceremonies, infusing each moment with a smell memory of healing that stays with us long after a ritual has ended. A major benefit of using essential oils in ritual is that we will be receiving all the health benefits of aromatherapy on a consistent basis. The regularity of ritual can compound the therapeutic benefits of essential oils, ever improving our mental, physical, and spiritual wellness. However, it's crucial to note that not all essential oils are safe for frequent use. Some, like pennyroyal and nutmeg, are better reserved for exceptional circumstances. Here is my aromatherapeutic recipe for a personal protection ritual.

Praxis
Ritual Bath for Auric Protection

The following is a recipe for a weekly ritual bath blend to help in protecting your aura and energy.

You Will Need

- 1 drop frankincense (for protective divine energy plus weekly support of brain function)
- 1 drop vetiver (to ground and reset, plus provide some weekly stress relief)
- 1 drop juniper (for energy clearing, plus a weekly detoxification of the body)
- 1 teaspoon each carrier oil and salt

Directions

Drip the essential oils into a teaspoon of carrier oil, creating a 3 percent blend. Mix the oil blend into a ½ cup of salt, and then add to warm (not hot) bath water. When you enter the bath, take a moment to fully submerge your body in the water. Take a moment to sense that every part of you is being held by it. Then, find a comfortable position to begin visualizations guided by the experience of the essential oil aromas. Feel the weight of the vetiver grounding you, your body is fully supported. Feel the cleansing of the juniper reaching into all parts of your being, drawing out negative energy. Feel the frankincense connecting you to protective divinity.

Next, build up an auric shield through magickal intention and an energy shaping visualization—inhaling through the nose, visualizing pure white light entering the top of your head and filling your body and aura. See it becoming a sphere of protection that completely surrounds you. Focusing on the aroma of the frankincense and the divine white light that surrounds your body, see the outside surface of the sphere becoming stronger and more solid than pure light. A lasting protective shield forms all around you.

As you soak in the water, focus on the juniper essence, and visualize any negative energy being drawn out as sand-like grains that are ready to go down the drain. Taking notice again of the comforting weight of the vetiver, visualize your body supported by the earth, reground and center yourself. When you feel ready, pull the bath plug and acknowledge the grains of negativity, consciously visualizing them get pulled down the drain with the water that held you. It all leaves easily and completely; trust that it will be taken in lovingly by the earth and transformed into something beautiful.

Rites

Rites are rituals performed to celebrate a significant occasion or life event, such as the eight Pagan sabbats, handfastings, and eldering. Rites tend to be more involved than rituals: they might include several people and can take a significant amount of time to plan and organize. I like to use aromatherapy to set the general tone of a rite invoking the spirit of the event rather than focusing on any individual aspect.

 Praxis
Invoking the Spirit of Yule

For instance, by using essential oils that invoke characteristics of the sun, a Winter Solstice rite will feel truer to its purpose. My Winter Solstice rites are like a love letter to the sun. It is a celebration that honors the Yuletide's returning light. The spirit of the winter sun is warm, encouraging, bright, joyful, uplifting, and strong. Here's a diffuser recipe I might use to set the tone for this occasion.

You Will Need

- 5 drops clove bud essential oil
- 7 drops sweet orange essential oil
- 4 drops scotch pine essential oil
- Pottery tealight oil burner
- Water
- Beeswax candle and lighter

Directions

Fill the reservoir bowl of a pottery tealight oil burner with water and add the essential oils. Using a beeswax tea candle, light the flame that will heat the bowl of the burner to diffuse the blend into the environment. As the pleasing aroma diffuses into the atmosphere of the Winter Solstice rite, it invokes a sensory celebration of the sun's return. Immerse yourself in the welcoming warmth reminiscent of the sun's fiery energy in the clove bud oil. Experience the effervescent joy of the sun captured in the sweet orange oil. Feel the sun's robust strength and resilience embodied in the scotch pine oil.

With the aroma permeating the air, the sacred space has been mindfully scented, creating an ambiance conducive for the rite. Not only does this elevate the physical environment, but it also enhances the emotional resonance, inviting participants to connect more deeply with the spirit of the sun and the essence of Yuletide.

Spellcraft

The crafting and working of spells is an arcane fusion of ritual and meditation. It empowers us to consciously manipulate the energies around us to create positive outcomes. By seamlessly combining ceremonial practices with mental visualization, we're able to establish a mystical connection between our thoughts and the universe, harnessing its potential to bring about desired transformations. The work of spellcraft is intricate. Numerous methods and tools are available, and aromatherapy is a particularly effective one.

Essential oils serve not just as an aromatic addition, but as a potent amplifier to our magick and the spellcraft process. They heighten the energetic momentum and increase the power of the work, while also serving to prepare the mind, better enabling the practitioner to focus their intention. Spellcraft is also one of my specialties and I find that because of the variety and flexibility of aromatherapy, the two can be easily integrated.

Whether it's anointing a talisman with a specially prepared essential oil blend or filling the ritual space with fragrance, the methods we choose will directly affect the energy flow. To optimize the effectiveness of a spell, I think it is important to maintain a consistent theme across all aspects of spellcraft based on the spell's intention. In other words, the intention of the spell, the essential oils used, the method of their application, the ceremonial actions, ritual tools, and so on should all align within the context of the spell. Why? Because synergy in spellcraft adds power. When working with others, it's a good idea to have a discussion with everyone and everything involved to coordinate what both the process and the result will be. Not only will a check-in prevent any potential misunderstandings, it will also provide informed consent, which to me is essential.

Often, my role lies in crafting spells for others to personalize and cast. Consequently, the selection of oils and methods of use will heavily rely on the subjective element of the recipient. If a client came to me with the intention of casting a spell to find love, I might suggest essential oils such as rose or ylang-ylang, both renowned for their ability to open the heart chakra. However, the final decision lies with the individual who will ultimately benefit from the spell. The recipient must connect with the aromas and make the final selections based on their personal relationships with the oils, their intuition, and preferences. The spell must be unique to their energies to ensure the highest likelihood of success.

For the example that follows, I narrowed down the choices of essential oils to fit the spellcraft's intention. At this point, the recipient of the magick would need to be the one to finalize which essential oils to use in the blend. I wrote this spell as though the recipient is also the practitioner, but of course it doesn't necessarily need to be that way.

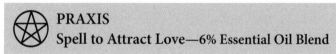

PRAXIS
Spell to Attract Love—6% Essential Oil Blend

This blend is to be used as an anointing oil for a candle magick ritual under a waxing quarter moon. The recipient chooses one oil per purpose. Use a total of 12 drops essential oils in 10 mL sunflower oil.

Oil Choices

Confidence building: Ylang-ylang, chamomile, or
   peppermint

Grounding: Patchouli, vetiver, or elemi

Love/heart opening: Rose, jasmine, or melissa

Joy inducing: Mandarin, lime, or bergamot

14 drops total of essential oils in 10 mL sunflower carrier
oil.

You'll also need

- A pink candle in a fireproof holder
- A candle scribing tool
- Index cards and a pen
- 10 mL sunflower oil as the carrier

Directions

First, the recipient chooses one oil per purpose. After that,
the spellwork continues.

1. Begin by clearing your space of any negative
   energy and ready it for sacred work. In preparation for the ritual, topically apply the blend
   to anoint your body. It can go anywhere, but do
   include the ankles, wrists, and over the heart.
   Always remember to check the phototoxicity
   risks of essential oils when they are being used
   on the body.

2. Write the following affirmations on an index card: *I commit to loving myself. I live my life as an expression of the divine love of the universe. I am surrounded by love, and I am worthy of its blessings.*

3. Take a pink candle and use a scribing tool to carve full hearts into the wax. Using the essential oil blend, anoint the candle starting from the middle and moving toward the two ends. As you do this, focus on your intent, to draw even more love into your life and in turn offer more love to the world.

4. Place your candle in its fireproof holder. As you light the candle, say your affirmation out loud. Believe in the words. Breathe in the power of the aromas. Let them permeate all aspects of your being. Meditate on their healing power for as long as feels right for you. When you feel ready, snuff the flame out and close your sacred space. Never leave a lit candle unattended.

5. Each evening, until the moon is full, anoint your body and your candle, repeating the ritual steps above.

6. On the last night of this spell, expand your consciousness with the fullness of the moon. Let your gratitude flow. Feel your intentions

being released to the universe and know that your desire is already coming to fruition. Surrender any need for control. Trust in the divine power within, and around you. When you are ready, blow out the candle flame with a "thank you" to fully close out the spell. Know that the energy of your work will continue to ripple out into the cosmos spreading and growing true love. So be it!

Visualization Guides

Feel your heart warming and allow yourself to know without any doubt that you deserve true love. Feel the love, respect, and gratitude you have for yourself and your body. Feel the joy that you bring to others and that they bring to you.

Allow yourself to let go of the fears that are holding you back from finding true love. Accept all love that lifts you up and celebrates you. Let it come easily into your life, and so it shall be.

Communing

Reaching out to the Divine is a profound act of magick. The distinction between the Divine, something being divine, and divine beings is subtle but significant. For me, "the Divine" is a term that refers to the overarching, all-encompassing aspect of divinity. I see it as a cosmic source, the ultimate interconnecting force, or the universal energy field from which all divinity springs. The Divine encompasses anything that is deeply spiritual, supremely good, and profoundly sacred. In other words, it represents the highest spiritual principle, the absolute truth that permeates the universe. When I describe something as divine, I'm usually attributing it with a spiritual or sacred quality. It could be an experience, a piece of music, a piece of art, or even an action that is so powerful it gives us a sense of connectedness to the ethereal realm. I identify divine beings as conscious entities with unique personified aspects of the Divine. They take many forms across different cultural, religious, and spiritual beliefs. Deities, angels, spirit guides, plant spirits, ancestors, and other ethereal creatures such as the Fae are examples of divine beings. In the broadest sense, communing with the Divine involves intentional and meaningful engagement with metaphysical and transcendent realms.

Essential oils like frankincense, myrrh, and sandalwood have long been believed to resonate with higher spiritual vibrations and promote deeper spiritual connection. Offerings of sacred aromas like these during prayer, meditation, or ritual work can also be seen as a sign of reverence and respect. The act of making offerings symbolizes our acknowledgment of the Divine, our gratitude for the blessings received, and our willingness to give something of value back to the cosmic order.

Another use for aromatherapy when communing with the Divine is to invoke specific divine beings. Depending on the deity or spiritual entity you wish to connect with, specific oils may be more appropriate than others. For instance, floral essential oils such as rose are often associated with love deities like the Greek goddess Aphrodite. Divine beings may also have complex personalities, or history that we want to commune with or acknowledge. Using essential oils can help us call to them in a very precise way and foster a particular connection with them. For example, when I want to invoke the Roman goddess Diana, I will usually call to her through one of her aspects: the Hunter, the Protector of Childbirth, or the Moon Goddess. The essential oils I use will have properties which align with that aspect's characteristics.

For the Hunter

Characteristics include confidence building, increasing focus, and clarity of mind. Rosemary essential oil would be great to support all these characteristics. Perhaps I would actively diffuse rosemary into my ritual space when drawing down the Hunter Goddess.

For the Protector of Childbirth

Characteristics include fertility, uterine health, and childbirth. A 13 percent essential oil blend would work well applied topically over the abdomen to anoint the body in preparation for ritual. Perhaps avocado oil would act as the carrier to invoke the essence of fertility. To represent uterine support, I might use geranium essential oil and I could call on the oil of rose as a patron of childbirth.

For the Moon Goddess

Characteristics include reflective, shines in the night, and awakening. Jasmine flowers scent night air, so their essential oil would be lovely as a way to honor the moon. I could drip the jasmine into a bowl of peppermint hydrosol intended to awaken the mind and reflect the moonlight.

I invite you to explore your different relationships with the Divine by channeling the spiritual energy inherent in all essential oils. When working with deities, try utilizing the methods of subjective exploration as a guide to help discover which oils and practices might resonate with them and why. Experiment and let your intuition guide you.

Divination

Like good friends, divination tools witness our struggles, share in our victories, and guide us when the path forward is shrouded in mystery. As we use them, we pour into them a piece of ourselves. Our energy transforms them from mere inanimate objects into instruments pulsing with our individual imprint. Just as we would use a diary or journal, we entrust these tools with our deepest thoughts, questions, and anxieties. But unlike a journal, divination tools will talk back, challenging our views, answering our questions, and soothing our doubts.

This interactive exchange of energy fosters a dynamic relationship and ongoing dialogue that grows more nuanced and profound with each interaction. The intimacy of this relationship is further heightened by the vulnerability that divination demands. The bond with our divination tools is not one-sided—over time, they respond to our openness by becoming attuned to the subtle shifts in our energies. As we grow and evolve, so do they, reflecting our changes back at us. Just like with essential oils, our relationships with our divination tools are an ongoing process of self-discovery, personal growth, and spiritual evolution. The more we use the tools of both divination and aromatherapy, the deeper we can delve into our psyche.

Just as I use divination methods to enhance my work with essential oils, I like to use aromatherapy to enhance my divination practices. My approach has two goals: open the receiving channels of the person doing the divination, and amplify the messages being sent from the Divine.

When I want to open up the diviner to be better able to receive and interpret messages, I like to start with a bit of light shadow work. The human experience is messy.

Prepare yourself for divination by identifying some of the personal baggage you may be carrying and addressing it. To be effective diviners, we need to be able to discern what messages are being received from a Divine consciousness and what is streaming from our own. Essential oils that best support shadow work are centering—black spruce, pine, and patchouli, for instance.

Once the diviner's unhelpful emotional accoutrement has been treated, I will look at how to increase their perception and insight. The goal is to be at our most receptive, which most often occurs when we're in a state of relaxed awareness. Receptivity can be encouraged and supported by essential oils that reduce anxiety but aren't sedating; they will help us to be attentive without being stimulated. Citrus oils can work wonderfully here, and my favorites are sweet orange and mandarin.

When I want to turn up the volume on communications sent from the Divine, I use tree resin oils. In my experience, essential oils that are distilled from tree resin specifically will carry the strongest divine signals, acting like a conduit between the cosmos above and the earth below. There are also several lovely essential oils distilled from other tree parts, like needles for pine oil, leaves for eucalyptus oil, and flowers for neroli. But resin essential oils such as elemi, frankincense, or myrrh, resonate with the liminal in a way that's perfect for divination amplification.

PRAXIS
Preparation for Divination

Remember, divination is not just about foreseeing the future, it's a profound conversation with the universe and your higher self. Enter that dialogue with an open heart, respect, patience, and curiosity.

You'll need

- ¼ teaspoon of olive oil
- 1 drop of an essential oil that helps you get centered (I recommend black spruce, pine, or patchouli)
- ¼ teaspoon of borage oil in a small bowl
- 1 drop of an essential oil that will help you get into a state of relaxed awareness (I recommend sweet orange, mandarin, or neroli)
- An ultrasonic diffuser or other active diffuser
- 9 drops of an essential oil that will amplify divine messages (I recommend elemi, frankincense, or myrrh)
- Your preferred ritual tool for divination—e.g., tarot cards, pendulum, or scrying bowl

Directions

1. Get centered. Find a comfortable sitting position and take three deep, grounding, breaths.

Settle into your body. Pour ¼ teaspoon olive oil into your palm and add one drop of your centering essential oil. Rub your palms together, cup your hands in front of your nose, then take three more deep breaths in through the nose and out through the mouth. Place one hand on your sternum and the other hand on your stomach. Breath and find your center.

2. Once you feel ready, begin some surface shadow work. Sort through any glaring issues that that might get in the way of correctly interpreting divine communications. Either move through it and let it go, or just put it aside until it can be thoroughly addressed. If you feel like you need a lot more support in that moment, consider waiting for a better time for divination. Alternatively, you could temporarily treat the root issues with aromatherapy, then put it aside so that you can more thoroughly examine it later.

3. Once you have completed the light shadow work, reground and center yourself. Take the small bowl holding ¼ teaspoon of borage oil and add 1 drop of the essential oil which will help you get into a state of relaxed awareness. Anoint your forehead with this blend over your third eye. Allow its calming and awakening energy to move through your mind, body, and spirit. Charge it to only allow messages

that are compassionate, helpful, and of the highest truth.

4. Start your diffuser using the 9 drops of divine signal boosting essential oil. Let the aroma swirl around you. Visualize yourself as part of a sacred tree, roots digging down into the soil from your feet, branches reaching up toward the cosmos from your hands, your body is like a conduit of divine communication. See and feel the tips of your roots and branches open up, focus on "tuning in" to the signals that you want to turn up the volume on.

5. Once you feel connected and ready, pick up your divination tool and begin your session of divination.

6. Remember that as witches, we must close the doors we open. Once you have completed your divination session, close any channels of communication that are not usually open throughout your day-to-day living.

7. Turn off your diffuser, close your eyes, and shift your focused attention to the protective aspects of the tree resin oil.

8. Once again, visualize yourself as the sacred tree. Close the tips of your roots and branches, to the point that feels safe and protected. Turn down the volume of your divine communication.

9. Sit in peace for a moment as part of the sacred tree. See yourself strong, grounded, and grateful. Zoom out your visualization to see and feel yourself sitting in a hushed and beautiful forest of sacred trees. There is so much wisdom and clarity here, and within you. Zoom out further, leaving the forest grove. Bring your awareness to the room you are in. Take a deep, grounding breath. Open your eyes, take another breath. Start to move your body and take a third breath, one of closure.

Chapter 8

Blending

Essential oils are a multi-faceted tool for creating an environment of well-being. I prioritize blending by oils' benefits, but I also try to create a pleasant fragrance experience. When blending based on aroma, it is important to first understand the characteristics of each oil so that you can create a blend that works for your desired effect. Although some aromas are instantly recognizable, the smell profile of an essential oil can vary depending on the growing conditions of its source plant. Variables include the plant's soil conditions, the climate, and the timing of harvest. Every batch of lavender essential oil is subtly different, but our familiarity with lavender's general aroma allows us to identify them all as lavender oil. The more we use essential oils, the more familiar we become with their aromas and the more accurate our interpretations of their fragrance.

Common Aroma Descriptions

When developing my sense of smell, I find it helpful to refer to aromatic descriptors that are often used in the perfume industry. Here is a list of keywords with their most defining qualities.

Amber: Resinous, gummy, warm, sweet

Animalic: Leathery, fur-like

Astringent: Penetrating, sharp, pungent

Balsamic: Rich, sweet, warm, earthy, woody

Bitter: Metallic green quality, without sweetness, sharp

Camphoraceous: Fresh, sharp, medicinal, clean, purifying

Citrusy: Citrus fruit-like, zesty, fresh, clean, bittersweet

Clean: Uncomplicated, fresh

Coniferous: Pine needles, woody, evergreen

Cooling: Feeling cold when inhaled, refreshing

Earthy: Mossy, moldy, forest floor like, dirt

Exotic: Intoxicating, heady, floral, tropical

Floral: Like a bouquet of flowers, perfumy

Fresh: Light, airy, clean, crisp

Fruity: Sweet, fresh, ripe, mouthwatering

Green: Foliage, moist leafy forest

Grassy: Freshly cut green grass

Harsh: Pungent, chemical, rough

Hay: Freshly cut hay, straw bales

Heady: Intoxicating, stimulating, sparkling, narcotic

Heavy: Intense, balsamic, almost suffocating

Herbaceous: Green, shrubby, camphoraceous, medicinal

Honey: Very sweet, syrupy, heavy

Leather: Pungent, smoky, sweet

Lemony: Zesty, lemon-like, crisp, clean

Medicinal: Camphoraceous, herbal, spicy

Minty: Cool, refreshing, peppermint-like

Mossy: Forest floor, green earth

Musty: Dusty, old papers, attic

Narcotic: Intensely intoxicating

Peppery: Spicy, stimulating, hot

Phenolic: Strong, disinfectant

Piney: Coniferous trees, evergreen

Pungent: Strong, sharp, intense

Resinous: Rich, deep, bittersweet

Rich: Penetrating, lingering, full

Smoky: Wood fire, char

Soapy: Detergent-like, lingering

Soft: Soothing, gentle, calming

Spicy: Hot, warm, exotic, peppery

Sweet: Sugary, candy

Warm: Comforting, like a hug

Woody: Tree bark, fresh cut wood

In general, contrasting scents tend to work well together and make for an interesting and dynamic aroma: sweet and smoky, spicy and floral, earthy and citrusy, as examples. You may find it helpful to use a fragrance wheel, a visual tool to aid perfumers and others who blend aromas searching for the perfect scent. Remember, it is also important to consider the ratio of each scent. Too much of one scent can overpower others and be overall too intense for some noses. The most successful aromatic blends are balanced.

Notes

To help us create an aromatic symphony, we can use aromatic notes. There are three categories of aromatic notes used in perfumery: base notes, middle notes, and top notes. The note of an essential oil is mostly determined by how quickly it evaporates, which makes it easy to find with the most basic research. Sometimes you will come across "cusp" notes such as base-middle and middle-top. The way in which you choose to use those can be informed by the context of your blend, what else is in it and what is needed to improve it.

Base notes are the foundation of a blend giving it depth and longevity. They tend to be heavier and more persistent than other scents, and they take the longest to evaporate. Popular choices for base notes include vetiver, patchouli, and sandalwood. Because of their lingering presence, recipes often use base notes most sparingly to achieve a balanced blend.

Middle notes evaporate more quickly than base notes, but not as quickly as top notes. They add more complexity and make a blend more robust. As the heart of a blend, they are often used in the highest concentration to bridge the gap between base and top notes. Some popular middle note oils include geranium, lavender, and cardamom.

Top notes are often the first impression of a blend. They evaporate the most quickly, so I try to choose top notes that can leave a lasting impression despite their fleeting fragrance. Popular top note oils include lemon, bergamot, and eucalyptus.

Notes in Magick

How fragrance is perceived will depend on the subjective element, but there are some guidelines for using aromatic notes to help influence a person's smell experience. Base notes often evoke a sense of groundedness. They can provide feelings of safety, balance, relaxation, and sureness.

Middle notes evoke a sense of openness. They can feel reassuring, encouraging, positive, and connected. Top notes evoke a sense of optimism. They can be energizing, stimulating, and leave us feeling refreshed.

Translated into magickal experiences, base notes are often used to invoke the element of earth. They particularly support the practice of centering and connect us to sources of spiritual wisdom. Middle notes can be used to invoke the elements of fire and water. They support wellness practices that tend to our inner landscape by connecting us to our individual emotional experience of the world, our behavior, and sources of healing and transformation. Top notes can invoke the element of air. They are clarifiers that support communication and divine inspiration. By adding precise intentions to the aromatic notes of a blend, we can further develop synergy, where the sum equals more than the parts.

Blending Methodology

Here's an overview my preferred method of essential oil blending:

1. Define the overall intention of the blend.
2. Break down the intention into its contributing factors.
3. Using your subjective element and essential oil profiles, assign aromatherapy treatments to support the intention's contributing factors.

4. Use perfumery notes and aromatic profiles to balance and help refine your blend.

5. Blend for your aroma preferences, determining the oil quantities through experimentation.

6. Choose method(s) of use.

Example of Self-Blending Scenario
In this example I create a Career Success blend for myself.

Step 1: Define the intention of the blend.
To increase my career enjoyment, recognition, and compensation.

Step 2: Break down the intention of the blend into the factors that contribute to its success.

- My career enjoyment is most affected by how much fun I am having and how stimulating the work is.

- My career recognition is most affected by the visibility of my work and client satisfaction.

- My career compensation is most affected by the popularity of my work and my energy level to do more.

Step 3: Prescribe oils to treat/support the contributing factors of my success.

Fun inducing: Bergamot, sweet orange

Stimulating: Basil, eucalyptus

> *Visibility:* Clary sage, vetiver
> *Client satisfaction:* Elemi, jasmine
> *Popularity:* Neroli, peppermint
> *Energizing:* Palmarosa, black pepper

Your confidence in choosing which oils to prescribe will grow with your knowledge base. As mentioned before, aromatherapy in magick is all about relationship building between you and your oils. When learning about oils, gather information from many different sources. Gather data from scientific research papers, books, classes, observations, and your subjective element. The more you know your oils, the easier they are to use.

Step 4: Add in perfumery notes and aroma profiles to my list of essential oil options to help me refine and focus the blend.

Fun inducing
> *Bergamot:* Top note—soapy, citrusy, clean
> *Sweet orange:* Top note—citrusy, fruity, sweet

Stimulating
> *Basil:* Top note—green, clean, rich
> *Eucalyptus:* Top note—camphoraceous, medicinal, cooling

Visibility

> *Clary sage:* Middle note—astringent, herbaceous, floral

> *Vetiver:* Base note—floral, smoky, sweet

Client satisfaction

> *Elemi:* Base note—woody, herbaceous, bitter

> *Jasmine:* Middle note—exotic, balsamic, floral

Popularity

> *Neroli:* Middle note—floral, bittersweet, heady

> *Peppermint:* Middle note—minty, cooling, sweet

Energizing

> *Palmarosa:* Middle note—honey, heavy, fruity

> *Black pepper:* Middle note—woody, animalic, spicy

Step 5: It's time to start blending.

My goal is for the end product to smell balanced and enjoyable while retaining the desired therapeutic benefits for my mind, body, and spirit.

One important note: Start by creating a few test blends using small amounts of oil so you can get the proportions right before committing to a full-sized batch. It will take some trial and error to find the perfect combination for your scent blend, but don't be afraid to experiment. It can also help to let your test blend variations rest at least overnight. When given sufficient time to meld, the harmony in a blend can be much improved.

Continuing with the example, I want my blend to use one essential oil from each of the six factors that contribute to my career success and for my blend to smell yummy. By comparing the list of oils from step 4, I can make educated estimates of which six oils might work best together. With some small-batch experimentation using varying oil quantities and ratios, I land on the following recipe.

Recipe: Dree's Career Success Blend
—100% essential oil
20 drops elemi
10 drops vetiver
10 drops black pepper
10 drops peppermint
10 drops basil
15 drops bergamot

Step 6: Use this blend.
The final step of this blending technique is to design the magickal methods of use. I chose to make a 100 percent essential oil blend with no carrier so that I could change the way I use it as needed. There are endless options for magickal methods of use, limited only by our imagination. Here are just three examples of how I could use this blend.

Sun-day Candle Magick

The added intention of this weekly ritual is to invoke the power of the sun to bring blessings of increased energy, visibility, and preparedness for the work week ahead. This practice aims to foster a sense of readiness and prosperity in both professional and personal aspects of one's life.

Carve a sun symbol into a gold altar candle. Light the candle each Sunday morning and add a drop of the Career Success blend into the melting wax under the flame. Then spend time in meditation visualizing a full yet manageable client roster, envisioning oneself and clients thriving in abundance, and feeling deeply connected and prepared for the work of healing.

Waxing Moon Dance Party

The added intention of this monthly ritual is to shake off any accumulated stress from the past month and recharge in the moonlight. A bumpin' playlist of good-time tunes is essential.

Use an ultrasonic diffuser to fill a room with the fragrance of the Career Success blend. Turn down the lights, turn up the music, and dance like no one is watching! Call in the empowering energy of the waxing moon and free yourself from self-limiting thoughts. Fearlessness grows with every shake of that booty, followed by your unstoppable success.

Penny Planting

The added intention of this spellcraft is to nurture the growth of financial resources. Like a seed of a money tree, the penny is planted in the earth accompanied by a prayer for abundance.

Take a penny and place it into a small dish of vinegar with a drop of the Career Success blend. The penny is soaked until it becomes shiny and beautiful, after which it is planted in soil. To set and maintain the spell, water the penny seed with a cup of water mixed with a drop of the blend. Visualize the money tree thriving, your bank balance increasing, and a clear path to financial freedom.

Blending For Others: An Example

Making assumptions about anything is usually ill-advised. But when helping others explore magickal aromatherapy, drawing probable conclusions is a necessary place to start. With so many options available, you will need to narrow down the field before beginning a full assessment of a client's subjective element. First, learn from the client what is needed, what is not needed, and what their vision is. Using your essential oil profile knowledge, from there you can make informed decisions and educated estimates on what will likely be the best aromatherapy options. Your selection of essential oils would then be introduced to the client for an assessment of their subjective element. In the following example, I have added space for this in step 3.

A quick reminder that before creating aromatherapy for anyone other than yourself, health risks and possible contraindications should be discussed and recorded on an intake form.

The Steps

In the following example, the client has no health conditions, no allergies, and no sensitivities. She has used essential oils in the past without any issues and doesn't have any particular likes or dislikes. She seeks aromatherapy to enhance her solitary full moon rites that are performed on a beach, and she doesn't work with any specific pantheon.

Step 1: Define the intention of the blend.

To awaken intuition and commune with the divine full moon.

Step 2: Break down the intention of the blend into the factors that contribute to its success.

- She worships the full moon as Goddess because it resonates with her inner divinity, helping her honor and worship herself.
- She has a hard time trusting her wisdom, which disconnects her from her intuition.

Step 3a: Initial essential oil selections

These are the conclusions drawn to narrow down the options.

Jasmine: Deep floral aroma, sacred to the moon

Frankincense: Resinous aroma, facilitates communication with the Divine

Peppermint: Fresh menthol aroma, awakening

Elemi: Resinous floral aroma, facilitates communication with the Divine

Clary sage: Herbaceous floral aroma, opens psychic channels

Ylang-ylang: Sweet floral, honors the divine feminine within

Now, her subjective element can be assessed with these six essential oils. She will smell and experience them, providing direct feedback for each.

Jasmine: Too sweet and flowery, remove.

Frankincense: Negative association from childhood spiritual trauma, remove.

Peppermint: Invokes the brightness of a full moon, keep.

Elemi: She enjoys the aroma, keep.

Clary sage: It's bright and awakening, and has a positive association with her mother, keep.

Ylang-ylang: "eww!" remove.

At this point, the number of options in her blend has been reduced to three. There are two paths moving forward: continue to introduce more essential options to analyze or proceed to step 3b using only these three essential oil options. For this example, we will keep it simple with the three oils.

Step 3b: Prescribe oils to treat/support the factors that contribute to the success of the blend.

> *Honor the divine feminine within and around:* Clary sage
>
> *Heighten psychic channels:* Clary sage
>
> *Improve self-trust:* Elemi

Step 4: Add perfumery notes and aroma profiles to the list of essential oil options to help refine and focus the blend.

Honor the divine feminine, within and around

> *Clary sage:* Middle note—woody, herbaceous, slightly floral
>
> *Heighten psychic channels*
>
> *Clary sage:* Middle note—woody, herbaceous, slightly floral
>
> *Improve self-trust*
>
> *Elemi:* Middle note—peppery, balsamic, evergreen

Step 5: It's time to start blending.

In step 3b, we went from three to two essential oils. Fantastic! A quality essential blend does not need to involve multiple oils with multiple notes. It only needs to feel balanced to the user, be enjoyable to use, and achieve the aromatherapeutic goals. After some small-batch trial and error, the following recipe is established.

Recipe: Client's Full Moon Rite Blend
—100% essential oil
10 mL clary sage
7 mL elemi

Using This Blend

The final step of this blending technique is to design the magickal methods of use. Taking the time to evaluate, customize, and connect an individuals' essential oil blend to familiar spiritual practices can help them get the most out of their aromatherapy. On the other hand, introducing new ideas adds a magick of its own. For this example, a discussion with the client led to two suggestions: a moon mister (super portable) and a moon water bowl (not as portable). The personal mister spray bottle is unassuming to prying eyes when doing magick in public places, and the essential oils can be absorbed through the nose and skin without being topically applied in a carrier oil, which is nice when at a sandy beach. The falling mist is also a fabulous visualization aid that can lend an empowering and invigorating feel. In the moon water bowl, she could add sea water at the beach, which is a lovely way to integrate the natural environment into the ritual. Reflective of the moon, the bowl would be great for scrying. A cool compress dipped in a moon bowl is an excellent visualization aid for stillness. It can feel grounding, quieting, and reverent.

Both a mister and a compress will likely, however, expose the Full Moon Rite blend to the client's skin, so it will need to be diluted in a carrier. In this case, the carrier must be distilled water, which means it will also need the appropriate amount of dispersant.

- *~ 3% Moon Mister:* 26 mL distilled water, 20 drops of polysorbate 20, 18 drops of Full Moon Rite blend. This will go into a 30 mL fine mist spray bottle and labeled. On the label is the name of the blend, the dilution, the ingredients, and the soonest expiration date of all contents.
- *~ 3% Moon Water Bowl:* 900 mL distilled water, 25 mL polysorbate 20, and 25 mL Full Moon Rite blend. This blend will go into a liter bottle and labeled. The quantity is probably large enough for 4 to 8 Full Moon bowls.

I would then provide the client with a silver bowl, a 100 percent organic USA unbleached cotton cloth, and some visualization guides as a printout or audio recording. Here are two examples.

Moon Mist Visualization Guide

Face the Moon and spray the mister above, around, and above you again. See the moon reaching down to meet you, filling the thousands of misty droplets with its light. Feel them gently fall upon you and fill your spirit. Take three deep breaths through the nose and experience the aromas. Feel the elemi clearing the pathway of divine communication, trust that connection. Feel the clary sage resonate with the divine feminine above you, and within you—your goddess self.

Moon Bowl Visualization Guide

Lift the bowl to the sky and feel the elemi reaching to the divine moonlight, drawing it down. Lower the bowl to see the light dancing on the water. Experience the aromas. Place your cloth in the bowl, fill it with water, gently wring it out, and hold the compress over your third eye. Feel it awaken your inner sight and activate your learned wisdom, strengthening your intuition.

Blending with a Pendulum

For many purposes, including divination and healing, a pendulum can be a powerful tool. Pendulum dowsing is also an effective way to create custom essential oil blends for spiritual use. Having access to a plethora of essential oils is an incredible gift and privilege that can also be overwhelming. Pendulum blending can be a fun way to take the pressure off our decision-making and leave it to fate.

I use my pendulum to create blends to either serve a specific purpose that I have clearly defined, or to serve a purpose that I may be consciously unaware of. For instance, I might ask it for a blend to help me meditate, or to help me commune with the oak tree in my backyard. Alternatively, I might ask it for a blend to help support the overall wellness of my mind, body, and spirit in that moment.

This technique doesn't necessarily require owning a large variety of oils. If the essential oils you have access to are owned by someone else (such as your professional aromatherapist), I recommend using your pendulum by running it over the essential oil entries in your grimoire. That way you can just take an ingredients list to your aromatherapist and have them blend it for you.

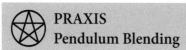

PRAXIS
Pendulum Blending

This technique is a great skill-builder. Using pendulum divination with aromatherapy blending can yield impressive results while building trust and confidence in the power of both.

You'll need

- Several different essential oils (or your aromatherapy grimoire)
- A pendulum

Directions

1. Start by selecting several oils that you already know and enjoy. Alternatively, use the essential oil profiles written in your grimoire.

2. Ground and center yourself. Connect to your pendulum and communicate what you need the pendulum to do. For example, "I need you to select three essential oils for a diffuser blend to help me commune with the backyard oak tree, please."

3. Establish how the pendulum will communicate yes and no.

4. One at a time, present each essential oil to your pendulum. Hover it over each oil and ask it for yes/no feedback, e.g., "Should this oil be included in today's blend to help me commune with the oak tree?"

5. Repeat, hovering over each of the oils until the pendulum has identified which to use in your blend. It's possible that more than three oils will be identified. In that case, take those selections and do a second pass over just those oil options.

6. Once the ingredients have been finalized, it's blending time. Decide how much of each oil to add to the blend based on your intuition and fragrance preferences.

7. When the blend is complete, offer a prayer of intention to infuse them with your spiritual energy and purpose.

8. Open your grimoire and journal any communique from the pendulum or oils. Include any feelings or impressions that arose during the blending process.

Commercial Blends

As a professional aromatherapist, my cabinet is a treasure trove of essential oils. I am lucky to have a rich tapestry of scents at my disposal, but if I were not in this profession, my collection would be much more modest. Most people need only a handful of essential oils supplemented with a few carrier oils and hydrosols. A seemingly limited collection of three to five essential oils can still meet a wide range of both magickal and mundane needs, but there's no denying that a smaller selection might pose certain aromatic constraints. This is where commercial blends can really shine. A well-crafted commercial blend can encompass a wide spectrum of scents, providing complexity and depth that individual oils might lack. Integrating a couple of these into a home collection can dramatically enhance its versatility, allowing for a more diversified exploration of aromatherapy's boundless potential.

The first thing to remember about commercial blends is that we probably won't know the origins of each essential oil in it. Unless the company you are buying from can provide explicit information about every ingredient in their blends, you might be supporting something that would normally constitute one of your ethical deal-breakers. For the sake of argument, let's assume that issue has been addressed and you feel good about using them.

One of the best things about commercial blends is that they have been professionally blended to smell awesome! Yummy fragrance is much easier to achieve when using large quantities of essential oils and the companies that create them are highly motivated to make aromas that appeal to many different people. My favorite thing about commercial blends is that they often include essential oils that would be prohibitively expensive to buy on their own (unless buying by the drop). These blends enable us to reap the benefits of several essential oils without needing to own them individually.

Commercial essential oil blends often have intention-based names like Inspire, Passion, or Energize. They are marketed to give people the idea that when they buy these oils, they will invite that specific feeling or quality into their lives. For example, a blend named Joy suggests that using it will bring more happiness to whomever uses it. Companies can objectively create these blends to affect our physiology in specific and therapeutic ways. To continue the example, a Joy blend might increase serotonin, reduce anxiety, and awaken the senses. But we know that the way each person experiences scent is subjective and unique. It's possible that the aromas that evoke pure joy in one person might smell like childhood trauma to someone else.

Choosing a Commercial Blend

When choosing a commercial blend to purchase, I recommend simply ignoring the name, because it only limits the potential. Focus on the contents and your experience of its aromas. Free it from the constraints of how it has been marketed. In situations where a commercial blend cannot be sampled, read through the ingredients and make educated guesses of how it might smell. Just to be clear, you'll never know for sure if you'll like a blend until you smell it, but the list of ingredients can help you decide on how it might be useful.

If I pick up a bottle called "Joy" and the ingredients listed were the essential oils of orange, patchouli, rose, lime, and bergamot, I would objectively expect this would indeed increase my happiness through its physiological impact...but what else might it do? After smelling its aroma, perhaps I'd start to feel playful and childlike. This tells me that this Joy blend would also be a beautiful offering to leave on my altar for the Fae folk. Perhaps the aroma would spark a nice smell memory, like playing in a park with my sibling as carefree children. It also tells me that Joy might work well for spellcraft intended to support my sibling through difficult times. I could attribute some magickal associations to the contents of Joy and note that it would be an incredible choice to accompany rites of union. It would be perfect to include a handfast-ing ceremony under the Solstice Sun.

Again, essential oils are complex and multifaceted, providing endless opportunities for inspired uses. While a commercial blend isn't exactly a custom blend, it can be just as good—or even better.

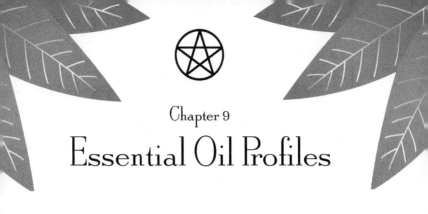

Chapter 9

Essential Oil Profiles

While the fragrances of essential oils and the metaphysics of aromatherapy are up for interpretation, their therapeutic characteristics are undebatable. Much of the healing power within these magickal substances lies in the science of their complex compositions. Essential oils are composed of natural chemical constituents, typically ranging from 100 to 400 different compounds in a single variety. Each oil's unique blend of chemical compounds gives it distinct properties that affect our physiology. The terpenoid compounds in essential oils can be broadly categorized into two types: hydrocarbons and their oxygenated derivatives.

Each chemical compound contributes to the overall therapeutic profile of an essential oil and works on many different levels. The intricate interplay of nature and chemistry in these precious drops of plant medicine will never cease to be amazing.

The Hydrocarbons

The two most prevalent families of hydrocarbons are monoterpenes and sesquiterpenes. Monoterpenes, which include compounds like limonene, pinene, and myrcene, are the most common group of terpenes found in essential oils. These hydrocarbons possess a diverse range of healing properties, and I consider them versatile protectors. Limonene, for example, is prevalent in citrus oils like lemon or sweet orange and is known for its uplifting properties. Pinene is most found in oils from trees such as pine and eucalyptus and is known to promote alertness and memory retention. It's also a powerful bronchodilator, helping to clear airways and making it beneficial for respiratory issues.

Sesquiterpenes, the deep healers, include compounds such as cedrene, azulene, and farnesene. Sesquiterpenes are generally found in lower concentrations than monoterpenes but their effects often occur on a deeper, emotional level. For example, cedrene, found in cedarwood oil, has a warm and grounding aroma that elicits a sense of profound connectedness. It promotes relaxation by stimulating the release of melatonin, a hormone that regulates sleep-wake cycles. Azulene is present in oils such as German chamomile and blue tansy, giving them their characteristic deep blue color. Azulene is a powerful anti-inflammatory and skin-soothing agent, excellent for calming eczema or irritations. It also evokes trust and helps cool our emotions, making it easier to communicate or accept hard truths.

Although monoterpenes and sesquiterpenes form only a part of the vast chemical universe contained in essential oils, they offer a fascinating glimpse into how these oils work on a molecular level.

Oxygenated Derivatives

Now, let's take a look at the oxygenated derivatives. These are found in essential oils as alcohols, esters, aldehydes, ketones, and phenols, among other forms. Alcohols are often characterized by their pleasant, uplifting aromas. Menthol is the primary component of peppermint oil and is an alcohol responsible for the oil's cooling sensation. It's often used for its analgesic properties to ease muscle pain and headaches.

Esters are known to alleviate stress, promote sleep, and support skin health. Linalyl acetate is an example found in high concentrations in lavender essential oil that can act as a mild sedative.

Aldehydes are generally recognized by their strong scents and potent antimicrobial properties. Cinnamon bark oil has a high amount of cinnamaldehyde which gives the oil its characteristic spicy aroma and germ-killing reputation.

Although ketones have a wide range of healing properties, some can be neurotoxic when used in high amounts or over long periods of time and should therefore be approached with caution. For example, camphor has a strong, penetrating aroma that is predictably found in camphor essential oil. It is often used for its invigorating and decongesting properties.

Phenols often have intense and herbaceous aromas. Due to the increased potential for skin irritation, they too should be used with caution. The phenol carvacrol contributes to the immune boosting quality of oregano and thyme oils.

Making Use of Chemotypes

To get the most out of an essential oil experience, it pays to take the time to select the best oil for the job. We want their therapeutic effects to be precise. Knowing about chemotypes can help us make choices that are better informed. Chemotypes refer to plants of the same species that produce essential oils with significantly different chemical compositions due to environmental factors such as climate, soil quality, and sunlight. Understanding chemotypes can also help us identify what compounds are present that might pose a safety issue.

For instance, rosemary (*Rosmarinus officinalis*) has several chemotypes:

> *Rosmarinus officinalis CT cineole* is high in oxides and is known for supporting respiratory health and aiding in mental clarity.

Rosmarinus officinalis CT verbenone is higher in verbenone and is reputed for its skin-regenerating properties.

Rosmarinus officinalis CT camphor contains more camphor and has a warming effect, making it ideal for soothing sore muscles and joints.

The scientific side of aromatherapy objectively studies essential oils and measures their physiological healing properties, but we can't measure magick. We can only observe what happens when we use essential oils in a spiritual way and draw some conclusions based on our logic and intuition. Th ere is a rich history of incredibly magickal folks that have done this and recorded their findings for us to learn from. There is absolutely noth-ing wrong with using essential oils in magick based on the associations assigned to them by someone else, as long as they resonate with you. If you read something that tells you ginger oil is the perfect choice to honor Jupi-ter and that makes complete sense to you, of course you should use it to honor Jupiter. However, I think it can be really beneficial to determine some of our own metaphysical associations and correlations.

For example, let's consider some magickal possibilities for ginger essential oil. First, ginger (*Zingiber officinale*) is a rhizome, a type of root deeply entrenched in the embrace of the earth. Naturally, aligning ginger with the power of the earth element makes perfect sense. Some traits that I associate with this element are steadfastness, stillness, and the physical realm. Similarly, ginger exudes a sense of stability that is grounding and makes us feel safe. But we can't stop there at its tranquil facade.

Some of ginger essential oil's physiological healing properties are that it is a stimulant, it increases blood flow, it gets things moving. We also know that ginger is spicy, possessing a fiery spirit that sets it ablaze with captivating passion. I associate the element of fire with motivation, activity, and transformation. Ginger would be a great choice to invoke the traits of fire.

Ginger essential oil is renowned for its therapeutic effect on the digestive system, connecting it to the solar plexus chakra, which is related to our self-worth and confidence. This association leads me to wonder what forms of empowering divinity might resonate with the essential oil. Perhaps an empowering crystal or gemstone such as carnelian would pair well with it.

To delve deeper into its mystical aspects, you might choose to go on a plant medicine journey with ginger essential oil (see chapter 6). Another option is using a pendulum to gather some direct feedback from it. Refer to your grimoire and make some magickal associations based on what you already know about ginger, adding to your notes as more possibilities are discovered. The only "wrong" correlation is one that has not been carefully considered. I invite you to view other people's associations and correlations as suggestions, not facts. Take the time to discover what resonates with you and trust your discernment.

55 Essential Oil Profiles

In this section is a list of essential oil profiles compiled from various sources including my personal experiences. It's a collection of professional consensuses regarding the general characteristics and properties of essential oils. This list is incomplete and is intended as a starting point for your own data collection.

Angelica Root
(*Angelica archangelica*)
Phototoxicity risk

Relieves/Combats: Cold and flu, viral infections, rheumatism, arthritis, physical fatigue, stress-related conditions

Promotes/Improves: Fortifying, strengthening, immune boosting, intimacy and closeness, inspiration

Metaphysical associations: Divine relationships, angelic ethereal realm, divination, energy cleansing, protection, prayer

Australian Sandalwood
(*Santalum spicatum*)

Relieves/Combats: Coughs, sore throats, respiratory issues, skin conditions and scarring, urinary tract infection, vaginal infections, insomnia, anxiety, nervous tension, exhaustion, depression

Promotes/Improves: Euphoric, elevating, opening, confidence, compassion, understanding, rejuvenating, aphrodisiac

Metaphysical associations: Divine connections, meditation, visualization, spiritual truth, grounding and centering, consecration

Basil
(*Ocimum basilicum*)
Avoid during pregnancy

Relieves/Combats: Muscular spasms, digestive issues, menstrual cramps, headaches, stress-related conditions, exhaustion, anxiety, fear, depression

Promotes/Improves: Focus, calm, strengthens mental functions, sharpens senses, clarity, nerve fortification, lactation, circulation

Metaphysical associations: Brings success and prosperity, psychic defense, protection, First Harvest (Lughnasadh)

Bay Leaf
(*Laurus nobilis*)
Can be a skin irritant

Relieves/Combats: Aches and pains, circulatory conditions, respiratory infections, digestive issues, colds and flu, nervousness, fatigue

Promotes/Improves: Liver and kidney tonic, stimulating, inspiration, self-esteem, courage, intellect, fortitude

Metaphysical associations: Divine wisdom, protection, energy shielding, divination, spiritual leadership

Bergamot
(*Citrus bergamia*)
Phototoxicity risk

Relieves/Combats: Infections, fevers, indigestion, depression, tension, insomnia, fear, emotional crisis, grief

Promotes/Improves: Heart opening, balancing, emotionally healing and stabilizing, motivation, happiness

Metaphysical associations: Fae folk, luck and good fortune, love magick, sun energy, illumination, youthfulness

Black Pepper
(*Piper nigrum*)

Relieves/Combats: Aches and pains, digestive problems, circulatory conditions, chills, exhaustion, mental blockages

Promotes/Improves: Reprogramming mental state, moving forward, nervous system tonic, endurance, courage, alertness, concentration

Metaphysical associations: Protection, severs unwanted attachments, manifestation, justice work, banishments, consecration

Black Spruce
(*Picea mariana*)

Relieves/Combats: Feelings of defeat, respiratory issues, sinus congestion, arthritis, rheumatism, stiff muscles and joints, stress-related issues

Promotes/Improves: Invigorating, motivating, adrenal system tonic, stress relief, inner peace, understanding

Metaphysical associations: Divine relationships, brings insight, Universal connectedness, grounding and centering, forest spirits

Cannabis
(*Cannabis sativa* L.)

Relieves/Combats: Anxiety, depression, inflammation, stress-related conditions

Promotes/Improves: Circulation, calming, energizing, harmonizing

Metaphysical associations: Green spirit energy, divination, protection from unwelcome spirits, fertility, spiritual growth

Cardamom
(*Elettaria cardamomum*)

Relieves/Combats: Fatigue, hopelessness, digestive issues, scalp conditions, sore muscles Promotes/Improves: Aphrodisiac, emotionally warming, comforting, uplifting, passion

Metaphysical associations: Sex magick, grounding, invokes playfulness, Summer Solstice (Litha)

Cinnamon
(*Cinnamomum zeylanicum*)
Can be a skin irritant

Relieves/Combats: Infections, colds and flu, fevers, aches and pains, exhaustion, fatigue

Promotes/Improves: Circulation, aphrodisiac, emotionally warming, energizing, joy

Metaphysical associations: Friends and family, inspiration, protection, Midwinter (Imbolc), spiritual leadership, purification, consecration

Clary Sage
(*Salvia sclarea*)
Avoid during pregnancy

Relieves/Combats: Menstrual symptoms, menopausal symptoms, aches and pains, muscular fatigue, excessive perspiration, headaches, scalp conditions, loss of concentration, insomnia, nervousness, depression, anxiety

Promotes/Improves: Memory, mentally stimulating, emotionally balancing, euphoric, reassuring, inspiration, supportive in times of change

Metaphysical associations: Psychic dreaming and clarity, divination, awakens intuition, moon energy, divine feminine

Clove Bud
(*Eugenia caryophyllata, Syzygium aromaticum*)
Can be a skin irritant

Relieves/Combats: Aches and pains, infections, toothaches and gum disease, muscular fatigue, nausea, stomach cramps

Promotes/Improves: Thyroid balancing, uterine tonic, immune boosting, memory, nervous system tonic, stimulating, breaking of unhelpful patterns

Metaphysical associations: Protection, hearth and home, transformation, rebirth, fire energy, Winter Solstice (Yule)

Copaiba
(*Copaifera officinalis*)

Relieves/Combats: Inflammation, anxiety, indigestion, skin conditions, aches and pains, insomnia, respiratory issues

Promotes/Improves: Immune boosting, nervous system tonic, balancing, mood-lifting

Metaphysical associations: Grounding and centering, ancestral healing, reassuring, meditation, daily devotions, prayer

Coriander Seed
(*Coriandrum sativum*)
Avoid during pregnancy

Relieves/Combats: Digestive problems, nervous tension, muscular fatigue, aches and pains, mental, emotional exhaustion

Promotes/Improves: Mentally invigorating, confidence, aphrodisiac, focused creativity, revitalizing, heals emotional trauma, detoxifying

Metaphysical associations: Spiritual awakening, letting go, transcendence, intuition, life force

Cypress
(*Cupressus sempervirens*)

Relieves/Combats: Swelling, gingivitis, hemorrhoids, congestive conditions, menstrual cramping, menopausal symptoms, respiratory conditions, grief

Promotes/Improves: Calming, increases objectivity, soothing, detoxifying, supportive in times of change, endurance

Metaphysical associations: Divine underworld, Hallow's Eve (Samhain), ancestors and descendants, drawing out, purifying, fortifying

Elemi
(*Canarium luzonicum*)

Relieves/Combats: Stress-related conditions, respiratory conditions, muscular fatigue, skin conditions, wounds, infections, exhaustion

Promotes/Improves: Lucidity, immune boosting, restorative, regenerative, sedative, focus, inner peace, balancing to nervous system

Metaphysical associations: Divine connections, harmony, meditation, universal oneness, heals disjunction and divisiveness

Eucalyptus
(*Eucalyptus globulus*)
Can lower blood sugar levels

Relieves/Combats: Respiratory conditions, headaches, colds and flu, fever, aches and pains, infections, high blood sugar, anger, overwhelm

Promotes/Improves: Oxygenation of blood, regenerative, stimulating, refreshing, increases intellectual capacity, balancing

Metaphysical associations: Divine communication, energy cleansing, spiritually awakening, centering, air energy

Frankincense
(*Boswellia carterii*)

Relieves/Combats: Mental fatigue, confusion, respiratory issues, infections, depression, stress, wounds and scars, urinary tract infections, anxiety, nervousness

Promotes/Improves: Brain function, soothing, uterine tonic, immune boosting, emotionally balancing, mentally fortifying, serenity, heals trauma

Metaphysical associations: Divine connections and communication, loosens blockages, severing ties to the past, meditation, awareness of breath

Geranium
(*Pelargonium graveolens*)

Relieves/Combats: Sore throat, menstrual symptoms, menopausal symptoms, hemorrhoids, neuralgia, skin conditions, depression, fatigue, emotional crisis, stress-related conditions, mastitis, anxiety

Promotes/Improves: Circulation, detoxifying, sedative, uplifting, balances and regulates hormones, regenerative, sensuality, fertility, calms and energizes

Metaphysical associations: Spring Equinox (Ostara), breaks negative thought patterns, communication, self-expression, balances passive and aggressive energy, ritual facilitation, nurturing

German Chamomile
(*Matricaria chamomilla*)

Relieves/Combats: Anger, depression, allergies, skin conditions, digestive issues, inflammation, aches and pains, menstrual conditions, menopausal symptoms

Promotes/Improves: Calming, releasing of emotions, soothing, opening, wound healing

Metaphysical associations: Communication, expressions of truth, letting go, supports nurturing bonds

Ginger
(*Zingiber officinale*)
Can be a skin irritant

Relieves/Combats: Muscular fatigue, aches and pains, congestion, colds and flu, sore throat, digestive issues, nervous exhaustion, jet lag

Promotes/Improves: Circulation, aphrodisiac, stimulating, warming, sharpens senses, communication, immune boosting, confidence

Metaphysical associations: Opens emotions, lifts unneeded fear, transformational rites, sex magick, purifying

Grapefruit
(Citrus paradisi)
Phototoxicity risk

Relieves/Combats: Water retention, muscular fatigue, stiffness, depression, colds and flu, headaches, nervous exhaustion, stress-related conditions

Promotes/Improves: Uplifting, motivating, detoxifying, lymphatic tonic, circulation, skin tonic

Metaphysical associations: Courage and confidence, joy, energy clearing, career support, moving onward and upward

Helichrysum
(Helichrysum italicum)
Avoid during pregnancy

Relieves/Combats: Aches and pains, bruising, wounds, respiratory congestion, indigestion, swelling, hemorrhoids, skin conditions

Promotes/Improves: Circulation, clarity, compassion, liver and pancreas stimulant, restorative, longevity and resilience, mental flexibility

Metaphysical associations: Illumination, acceptance, intuition, psychic dreaming, meditation, supports growth and evolution, decision making

Himalayan Cedarwood
(*Cedrus deodara*)

Relieves/Combats: Respiratory infections, congestion, urinary tract infections, scalp conditions, insomnia, stress, anxiety

Promotes/Improves: Sense of control, comforting, strength and resilience, focus, sedative

Metaphysical associations: Energy cleansing, grounding and centering, justice work, spiritual expansiveness, meditation, psychic communication

Hyssop
(*Hyssopus officinalis*)
Avoid during pregnancy/nursing; avoid epilepsy

Relieves/Combats: Cold and flu, respiratory issues, aches and pains, digestive spasms, sore throat

Promotes/Improves: Alertness and awareness, clarity, compassion, understanding, creativity, releasing emotional pain

Metaphysical associations: Energy clearing, divination, creating sacred space, universal oneness, meditation, centering

Jasmine
(*Jasminum grandiflorum*)
Avoid during pregnancy

Relieves/Combats: Menstrual symptoms, stress-related conditions, apathy, fatigue, insecurity, anxiety, depression, fear, personal blocks

Promotes/Improves: Confidence, aphrodisiac, uterine tonic, lactation, skin nourishing, mood balancing, uplifting, optimism, artistic expression

Metaphysical associations: Moon energy, love and trust, spiritual growth, intuition, gratitude, releases personal blocks, hope

Juniper
(*Juniperus communis*)

Relieves/Combats: Fluid retention, urinary tract infection, abdominal bloating, cramping, hemorrhoids, respiratory issues, hangovers, fatigue, eczema, congested skin

Promotes/Improves: Detoxifying, reviving, strengthening, circulation, nervous system tonic, memory

Metaphysical associations: Purifying, dispels malicious energy, protection, sacred space, auric cleansing, ritual baths, consecration

Lavender
(*Lavandula angustifolia*)

Relieves/Combats: Inflammation, infections, skin conditions, insomnia, nervousness, stress-related conditions, sunburn, cramps, headache, respiratory issues, sore throat, depression, irritability, worry, anger, anxiety

Promotes/Improves: Balance, nervous system strengthening, intimacy, overall health and well-being

Metaphysical associations: Meditation, abundance, sacred humility, cleansing, spiritual healing, psychic ability, intuition

Lemon
(*Citrus limon*)
Phototoxicity risk; can lower blood pressure

Relieves/Combats: Anemia, greasiness, viral skin conditions, high blood pressure, joint pain, throat infections, colds and flu, indigestion, fatigue, fear, emotional outbursts

Promotes/Improves: Circulation, liver tonic, uplifting, revitalizing, nervous system fortifying, immune boosting, detoxifying, cooling, communication

Metaphysical associations: Cleansing, protection, purifying, decision-making, motivation, inspirational, awareness

Lemongrass
(*Cymbopogon citratus*)
Phototoxicity risk; can be a skin irritant

Relieves/Combats: Inflammation, gingivitis, digestive issues, exhaustion, excessive perspiration, aches and pains, depression, headaches, fever

Promotes/Improves: Anti-fungal, uplifting, calming, insect repellent, astringent, invigorating, diuretic, focus

Metaphysical associations: Psychic ability, channeling, forgiveness, divination, celebratory, togetherness, repels bothersome entities

Lime
(*Citrus aurantifolia*)
Phototoxicity risk

Relieves/Combats: Digestive issues, sore throat, colds and flu, depression, lethargy, chronic fatigue, hopelessness

Promotes/Improves: Refreshing, uplifting, lymphatic tonic, detoxifying, immune boosting

Metaphysical associations: Clarifying, purging of negativity, inspiration, auric cleansing, abundance, protection, friendship

Mandarin
(*Citrus reticulata*)
Phototoxicity risk

Relieves/Combats: Digestive issues, nervous spasms, colds and flu, congestion, sleep disorders, tension, irritability, stress, grief, emotional shock

Promotes/Improves: Calming, comforting, harmonizing during pregnancy, sedative, lymphatic stimulant

Metaphysical associations: Inner child shadow work, nurturing, change and transition, nonjudgmental support

Melissa
(*Melissa officinalis*)
**Avoid during pregnancy;
can be a skin irritant; can lower blood pressure**

Relieves/Combats: High blood pressure, fear, grief, depression, anxiety, agitation, digestive issues, diabetes symptoms, inflammation

Promotes/Improves: Calming, trust building, regenerative, emotionally warming and opening, encouraging

Metaphysical associations: Protection, unity, acceptance, May Day (Beltane), love, hope, cycle of life/death/rebirth, divination

Myrrh
(*Commiphora myrrha*)
Avoid during pregnancy/nursing

Relieves/Combats: Gingivitis, skin conditions, infections, loss of appetite, arthritis, cough, sore throat, indigestion, hemorrhoids, loss of appetite, itchiness

Promotes/Improves: Revitalizing, fortifies the mind, nervous system tonic, focus, motivating, empowering, restorative, calms inflamed emotions

Metaphysical associations: Psychic ability, intuition, spiritual leaders and educators, meditation, divination, sacred space

Myrtle
(*Myrtus communis*)

Relieves/Combats: Respiratory issues, sinus infection, colds and flu, urinary tract infection, depression, insomnia, skin disorders, hemorrhoids, aches and pains, exhaustion

Promotes/Improves: Courage, uplifting, rejuvenating, balancing, confidence, immune boosting, stimulating

Metaphysical associations: Divine connections, truth and authenticity, love, protection through times of change, rites

Neroli
(Citrus aurantium)

Relieves/Combats: Anxiety, fear, inflammation, stress-related conditions, depression, insomnia, indigestion, sensitive skin and scarring, high blood pressure

Promotes/Improves: Calming, reassuring, overall skin health, joy, optimism, relaxation, aphrodisiac, inner peace, confidence

Metaphysical associations: Divine connections, centering, spiritual healing and repair, love, ritual baths, shadow work

Niaouli
(Melaleuca quinquenervia)

Relieves/Combats: Respiratory issues, colds and flu, muscular injuries, aches and pains, fatigue, headaches, confusion, exhaustion

Promotes/Improves: Invigorating, awakening, immune boosting, concentration, assertiveness

Metaphysical associations: Clarity, decision-making, spiritual purpose, protection from psychic attack

Palmarosa
(Cymbopogon martinii)

Relieves/Combats: Skin conditions and scarring, infections, muscular fatigue, stress, irritability, restlessness, insect bites, inflammation

Promotes/Improves: Reassuring, balancing, resilience, confidence, stimulating, cooling, overall skin health

Metaphysical associations: Meditation, self-love, moving forward, affirmations, auric cleansing, purpose

Patchouli
(*Pogostemon cablin*)

Relieves/Combats: Stress-related conditions, skin conditions, water retention, nervous exhaustion, depression, anxiety

Promotes/Improves: Insect repellent, regenerative, satisfaction, balancing, concentration, aphrodisiac, calming

Metaphysical associations: Fall Equinox (Mabon), sacred space, grounding and centering, meditation, gratitude, wisdom, earth energy

Peppermint
(*Mentha piperita*)
Avoid during pregnancy/nursing

Relieves/Combats: Fatigue, congestion, digestive issues, gingivitis, hot flashes, menstrual cramps, headaches, itching, aches and pains, nervousness, inferiority

Promotes/Improves: Energizing, warming and cooling, alertness, revitalizing, sharpens the mind, stimulating

Metaphysical associations: Prosperity, insight, humble aspiration, psychic development, protection, clearing, manifestation

Petitgrain
(*Citrus aurantium*)

Relieves/Combats: Anxiety, depression, inflammation, stress-related conditions, insomnia, indigestion, skin conditions

Promotes/Improves: Calming, reassuring, nervous system tonic, optimism, relaxation, aphrodisiac, inner peace, confidence

Metaphysical associations: Harmony, centering, trust, consecration, meditation, clarity

Ravintsara
(*Cinnamomum camphora*)
Avoid when nursing

Relieves/Combats: Respiratory issues, aches and pain, colds and flu, infections, fatigue

Promotes/Improves: Immune boosting, self-confidence, stimulating, focus, reinvigorating, stimulating, brain function

Metaphysical associations: Energy cleansing, clarity, healthy boundaries, conviction, decision making

Rose
(*Rosa damascene*)

Relieves/Combats: Menstrual symptoms, infertility, skin conditions and scarring, depression, anxiety, insomnia, stress-related conditions, grief, jealousy, disappointment, emotional trauma

Promotes/Improves: Hormone balancing, uterine tonic, emotionally opening, trust and love, compassion, aphrodisiac, confidence, satisfaction, uplifting

Metaphysical associations: Divine love, dissolves emotional blocks, wisdom, grounding and centering, deep healing, water energy

Roman Chamomile
(*Anthemis nobilis/Chamaemelum nobile*)

Relieves/Combats: Muscular spasms, fevers, menstrual cramps, skin conditions, insomnia, anxiety, nervousness, depression, stress-related conditions, digestive issues

Promotes/Improves: Emotionally balancing, replenishing, sedative, restorative, humility

Metaphysical associations: Dream states, calming to overactive energy centers, projection of healing, channeling

Rosemary
(*Rosmarinus officinalis*)
Can raise blood pressure; avoid epilepsy

Relieves/Combats: Fatigue, skin and scalp conditions, fluid retention, aches and pain, respiratory conditions, high cholesterol, colds and flu, headaches, stress-related disorders

Promotes/Improves: Brain function, adrenal tonic, cardiac tonic, uplifting, invigorating, circulation, concentration

Metaphysical associations: Psychic protection, drives out negative energy, will power, ambition, clairvoyance, centering, loyalty, ancestors

Sage
(*Salvia officinalis*)
Avoid during pregnancy/nursing; avoid epilepsy

Relieves/Combats: Hair loss, fluid retention, aches and pains, digestive issues, colds and flu, headaches, nervous exhaustion, stress-related conditions

Promotes/Improves: Overall health, attentiveness, regulates nervous system, uplifting, soothing, clearing, circulation

Metaphysical associations: Energy cleansing, trance states, shifts negativity, wisdom, spiritual awareness

Scotch Pine
(*Pinus sylvestris*)
Can raise blood pressure

Relieves/Combats: Aches and pain, muscular fatigue, infections, respiratory issues, sore throat, scalp conditions, exhaustion, anxiety, stress

Promotes/Improves: Circulation, refreshing, revitalizing, detoxifying, adrenal tonic, diuretic

Metaphysical associations: Divine communication, clearing, empathic protection, meditation, forest spirits, preparing sacred space

Sweet Fennel
(*Foeniculum vulgare*)
**Avoid during pregnancy/nursing;
avoid estrogen-dependent cancers**

Relieves/Combats: Digestive issues, menstrual symptoms, menopausal symptoms, fluid retention, fatigue, respiratory conditions

Promotes/Improves: Detoxifying, fertility, liver and spleen tonic, muscle-toning, aphrodisiac, calming, perseverance, courage

Metaphysical associations: Protection from psychic attacks, auric cleansing, handfastings, shadow work, awareness of truth, divination

Sweet Marjoram
(*Origanum majorana*)
**Avoid consistent long-term use;
can lower blood pressure**

Relieves/Combats: Aches and pain, spasms, numbness, menstrual symptoms, menopausal symptoms, headache, digestive issues, insomnia, stress-related conditions, anxiety, chronic fatigue

Promotes/Improves: Relaxing, comforting, longevity, willpower, comfort from loneliness and grief

Metaphysical associations: Trance states, ancestral wisdom, love, interpersonal connection, good fortune

Sweet Orange
(*Citrus sinensis*)
Phototoxicity risk

Relieves/Combats: Indigestion, depression, gingivitis, water retention, constipation, aches and pains, stress-related conditions, anxiety, insomnia, cold and flu

Promotes/Improves: Immune boosting, optimism, joy, uplifting, playfulness, creativity, emotionally warming

Metaphysical associations: Sun energy, self-awareness, harmonizing, friendship, generosity, abundance

Tea Tree
(*Melaleuca alternifolia*)

Relieves/Combats: Infections, wounds, scalp conditions, respiratory conditions, bites and stings, panic, emotional shock, headaches

Promotes/Improves: Immune booster, restorative, cleansing, centering, resilience and strength

Metaphysical associations: Clearing, consecration, banishment, warding protection, justice

Thyme
(*Thymus vulgaris*)

Relieves/Combats: Inflammation, sore throat, infections, colds and flu, respiratory conditions, aches and pain, muscular fatigue, lethargy, fear

Promotes/Improves: Circulation, energizing, motivation, brain function, resolve, confidence

Metaphysical associations: Divine masculine, purpose, protection, strength to recover, grounding, crossing over into the afterlife

Vetiver
(*Vetiveria zizanioides*)

Relieves/Combats: Stress-related conditions, circulatory conditions, aches and pain, restlessness, workaholism, physical exhaustion, irritability, depression, anxiety, fear

Promotes/Improves: Rejuvenating, immune boosting, balancing, comforting, nervous system tonic, harmonizing, stimulates red blood cell production

Metaphysical associations: Grounding and centering, energy shielding, spiritual wisdom, purpose, tranquility, journeying

Yarrow
(*Achillea millefolium*)
Can be a skin irritant; can lower blood pressure

Relieves/Combats: Inflammation, aches and pains, cramping, scarring, itching, high blood pressure, stress-related conditions, emotionally balancing

Promotes/Improves: Circulation, introspection, inspiration, awareness, understanding, moving through past hurt

Metaphysical associations: Shadow work, grounding, intuition, goal setting, discernment, meditation

Ylang-Ylang
(*Cananga odorata*)
Can lower blood pressure

Relieves/Combats: Stress-related conditions, high blood pressure, menstrual symptoms, menopause symptoms, fear, frustration, cramping, insomnia, anxiety, physical exhaustion, depression

Promotes/Improves: Aphrodisiac, circulation, security, serenity, deep relaxation, openness to change, positivity, creativity, understanding, euphoric

Metaphysical associations: Divine androgyny, love and trust, intuition, gratitude, body praise, sex magic

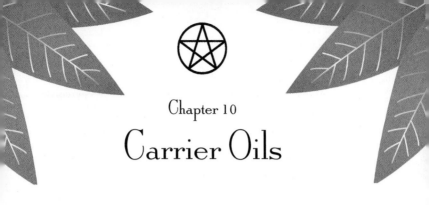

Chapter 10

Carrier Oils

Often, the carrier oil is seen as the unimportant medium that holds the important essential oils. Even the term "carrier oil" evokes a feeling of unimportance, as if it just carries the stuff that actually matters. However, I invite you to look at it this way, a 5 percent essential oil blend is 95 percent carrier oil—95 percent matters!

For magickal aromatherapy, I love to use carrier oils expressed from plants. Carrier oils extracted from plant parts share several traits with essential oils: both have therapeutic properties, magickal associations and correlations, and they also have countless uses for the mind, body, and spirit. Carrier oils also have their own inherent energy that to me feels a bit slower, less intense, less raring to go than essential oils. Despite their chill vibe, they each offer unique specialties that add power to our magick. When I make a magickal blend of aromatherapy, I try to imbue the carrier oil with my intention before adding the essential oils. That way, I am starting with a foundation that already has a focused and clear direction of healing.

Picking a Carrier Oil

When assessing the quality of carrier oils, some keywords we want to see on the label are Unrefined, Cold-Expressed, No Additives, and (ideally) Organic. The purity of an oil will determine whether it needs to be refined. Unrefined oils are so pure that they do not need to go through a process of refinement and, because heat degrades oil, they are always cold-press extracted. Cold-pressing is a form of oil extraction in which the origin plant matter is never heated above 81.9 degrees Fahrenheit, preserving its quality. When shopping for carrier oils, use the best—you deserve it.

I buy most of my carrier oils at the grocery store. In fact, it's highly likely that you have at least one good carrier oil in your kitchen cupboard. Even without essential oils, when infused with the power of your intention and the influence of your uniqueness, culinary carrier oils are perfect for impromptu mealtime magick. The next time you make a salad, charge that drizzle of olive oil with a magickal healing purpose. So mote it be absolutely delicious!

Dilution

As previously stated, pure essential oils should not come in direct contact with skin. For them to be safely diluted, they need to be thoroughly mixed with an oil-based carrier or suspended in a dispersant. When preparing an aromatherapy blend, we want the ratio of essential oil to its carrier to be safe and have optimal efficacy. Following, you'll find "cheat sheets" with key ratios and conversions for blending dilutions. It's important to note that the measurement "drops" is imprecise, as the viscosity and weight of an essential oil drop can vary significantly. For our magickal aromatherapy purposes, a close approximation is good enough.

When applying essential oils to a large skin surface area such as in a body massage, I recommend a blend of 1 to 5 percent essential oil in a carrier. However, reactive skin and sensitive areas like the face need a mild 0.5 to 1 percent essential oils in a carrier. This is also a good ratio for when working with children. When applying essential oils to a small skin surface area such as on the feet or a chakra point, a blend of up to 15 percent essential oil in a carrier would work.

Carrier Oil Profiles

Here are some commonly used carrier oils with generally accepted skincare benefits and my personal take on their metaphysical properties.

Apricot Kernel
Calming, restorative, ready for change

Apricot kernel oil is a bit of a hidden gem that's not as well-known than almond or coconut oil but just as spectacular. Rich in vitamins A and E, as well as omega-6 fatty acids, it's a real treat for all skin types. This oil is calming and gently nourishing, alleviating redness and inflammation. Apricot kernel oil is also restorative; it helps the skin regenerate, repairing the skin barrier and promoting the growth of healthy new cells. Spiritually, apricot kernel oil is associated with readiness for change. Just as the apricot tree naturally sheds the old and embraces the new, this oil symbolizes our own readiness to transform. It's like a catalyst, stirring us to shed old patterns and embrace the potential for growth and renewal. It's a wonderful oil to incorporate into spiritual practices when we're embarking on a new chapter in life.

Avocado
Nourishing, protective, fertility

Avocado oil is very nourishing to the skin. It's filled with nutrients, including vitamins A, B, D, E, and K, and abundant fatty acids such as oleic and linoleic acids. As a result, it has excellent moisturizing properties and is believed to boost collagen production, enhancing the skin's elasticity, and reducing signs of aging. Avocado oil is often associated with fertility, but the benefits are not limited to the physical realm. The larger, spiritual concept of fertility goes beyond reproduction; it can also be about creativity, growth, and abundance in all areas of life. Using avocado oil in our aromatherapy and magick can spark ideas, invite new projects, and foster positive energy. Just as the avocado tree brings forth its nourishing fruit, its oil encourages the cultivation of a full and rich life.

Borage
Stimulating, regenerative, communing with the Divine
Borage oil is stimulating in the sense that it can help boost skin health and vitality. Its high gamma-linolenic acid (GLA) content plays a key role in maintaining the structure and function of the skin. It boosts the skin's elasticity and overall integrity, giving it a rejuvenating effect. On the spiritual plane, borage is a plant of courage and consolation. It's an oil we can turn to when seeking spiritual guidance. Not only does its inherent energy offer optimism and encouragement, it also helps us channel messages from the Divine. This is the perfect oil to use when communing with the ethereal realm.

Castor
Relieving, reparative, independence
Castor oil is an incredible addition when doing bodywork and massage. It has a thick and tacky consistency,

so I suggest using it with an oil that has more slip. When applied topically, it can deeply penetrate the skin layers, stimulating the body's own healing mechanisms. It has a high content of ricinoleic acid and can reduce inflammation, soothing achy muscles. It's even thought to boost the lymphatic system, supporting our natural detoxifying process. In spiritual practice, castor oil can help foster self-reliance and personal strength. It emanates a vibration of independence. It's all about cultivating an attitude of self-sufficiency and believing in our abilities. The magick of castor oil empowers us to heal and thrive on our own terms.

Coconut
Protective, assuredness, generosity

Coconut oil is incredibly protective. This is largely due to its high content of saturated fats, primarily lauric acid, which is well known for its antimicrobial properties. Applying coconut oil to the skin can help form a barrier that wards against environmental and microbial threats. Spiritually, it is a potent symbol of generosity. Just think about the coconut tree, abundantly providing food, drink, and shelter. Coconut oil captures this energy and is ready to spoil!

Fractionated coconut oil has been processed to separate the solid fats from coconut oil. It remains in a liquid form and has no aroma, which often makes it the preferred option in aromatherapy. However, I feel like the fractionating process changes its spirit a bit. When working magick using the energies of innovation, decisiveness, or ambition, fractionated coconut oil is an ideal choice.

Evening Primrose
Restorative, nourishing, lunar connections

Evening primrose oil is particularly treasured for its high content of gamma-linolenic acid. It has the potential to improve skin health by restoring moisture and elasticity, making it a favorite in many skincare routines. A little goes a long way with evening primrose oil. It can be added to virtually any topical blend associated with intuition, emotions, and inner wisdom. Just as the moon goes through phases, we too experience cycles in our lives. Evening primrose oil can help us honor and navigate them. Its connection to lunar energy makes it an excellent tool for rituals related to the cycles in life, emotional healing, and the divine feminine.

Grapeseed
Balancing, protective, abundance

Grapeseed oil is known for its balancing effects, particularly on oily skin. It can help regulate the skin's natural oil production without clogging pores, leaving the skin feeling hydrated but not greasy. It's light and is easily absorbed, making it a favorite for massage and skin care. The spiritual side of grapeseed oil overflows with a bountiful energy. Think of how one tiny grape seed can produce an entire vine heavy with grapes. It's a beautiful symbol of the abundant nature of our universe. Working with grapeseed oil can assist in cultivating a mindset of prosperity and openness to the flow of abundance in our lives. Whether we're seeking to attract more love, health, or success, grapeseed oil can be a powerful magickal ally.

Hemp Seed
Protective, expansive, celebratory

Hemp seed oil is packed with linoleic acid, alpha-linolenic acid, and gamma-linolenic acid. These polyunsaturated fatty acids make it a skin super-hydrator while its regenerative antioxidants protect the skin from stressors. Spiritually, hemp seed oil promotes a sense of expansiveness. It can help us open up and be ready to embrace new ideas and perspectives. That type of energy also has a freedom to it that feels celebratory. Hemp seed oil reminds us to celebrate our journey, our growth, our victories—whether they're big leaps or small steps. A fantastic choice when working any magick to help channel a sense of gratitude and joy for all aspects of life.

Jojoba
Softening, calming, resilience

Jojoba oil is a bit of a superstar in the carrier oil world. While technically a wax, but its texture and composition are very similar to our skin's natural sebum making it a champion when it comes to skincare. It's packed with antioxidants and essential fatty acids that help soothe and nourish the skin, making it soft, supple, and healthy. The jojoba plant thrives in harsh desert conditions making it a symbol of adaptability and endurance. It resonates with resilience and the ability to not just survive but flourish under difficult circumstances. Incorporating jojoba oil into magickal practices can strengthen our spiritual core and enhance our capacity to weather life's challenges with grace.

Olive
Regenerative, reinforcing, wisdom

Olive oil is well-known for its regenerative properties. Its oleuropein and hydroxytyrosol content aids in the repairing of cells and warding off damage. Although it is powerfully replenishing, it is also very gentle, leaving sensitive skin soft and supple. As for its spiritual side, olive oil has been regarded as a symbol of wisdom for thousands of years across different cultures. In Greek mythology, for instance, the olive tree was sacred to the goddess Athena, the deity of wisdom and strategic warfare. Using olive oil in spiritual practices can be a beautiful way to tap into ancient divinity, to seek clarity, and to connect with your inner wisdom.

Rose Hip Seed
Regenerative, intense, passion

Rose hip seed oil has a ton of vitamin C, which makes it awesome for improving the health of any skin type and anti-aging skincare routines in particular. It has the ability to penetrate the deeper layers of the skin to stimulate collagen production, improving skin elasticity and firmness. With its potent regenerative qualities, it can even aid the healing of scars, burns, and stretch marks. Rose hip oil is intense in the best possible way. Energetically, it translates as passion. The rose flower has long been associated with love and passion, so this is an easy connection to make. Using rose hip seed oil in spiritual practices can help ignite an enthusiasm for life, deepen self-love, and heighten sensuality. Adding it to a facial oil blend and using it with positive affirmations would be a beautiful way to magickally magnify one's inner divinity. Shine bright, gorgeous!

Sweet Almond
Soothing, protective, inspiration

Sweet almond oil is a fan favorite for skin care. This lightweight oil is ultra-soothing, making it a wonderful choice for all skin types. It's loaded with vitamins and fatty acids that calm irritation and help with uneven skin tone. This lovely oil is also a defender. The vitamin E in sweet almond oil protects the skin from environmental stressors such as pollution and UV radiation. In magick, almond trees are often associated with newness and promise due to their early blossoming in spring. Sweet almond oil can therefore symbolize inspiration and awakening in spiritual practices. It offers a calming reminder that new beginnings are always possible, which can be particularly powerful when moving through challenging times.

Sunflower
Light, nourishing, solar connections

Although sunflower oil is light and nongreasy, it is luxuriously rich with vitamins A, D, and especially vitamin E. This potent antioxidant can help protect the skin from damage caused by free radicals. It's an excellent moisturizer that keeps skin hydrated, soft, and smooth. Sunflowers always turn toward the sun, following its path across the sky. Using sunflower oil in your spiritual practice can help you tap into this solar energy, its vitality, strength, and transformational fire. Naturally, sunflower oil is fabulous in rituals that involve sun energy, such as morning meditations or sun salutations. Anointing the solar plexus chakra with this oil will help activate our self-confidence and connect us to our growing personal power.

Essential Oil Dilutions

Carrier	1% EO	2% EO	3% EO	5% EO	10% EO
1 teaspoon (5ml, 1/6 oz)	1 drop	2 drops	3 drops	5 drops	10 drops
2 teaspoons (10ml, 1/3 oz)	2 drops	4 drops	6 drops	10 drops	20 drops
3 teaspoons (15ml, 1/2 oz)	3 drops	6 drops	9 drops	15 drops	30 drops
4 teaspoons (20ml, 2/3 oz)	4 drops	8 drops	12 drops	20 drops	40 drops
5 teaspoons (25ml, 5/6 oz)	5 drops	10 drops	15 drops	25 drops	50 drops
6 teaspoons (30ml, 1 oz)	6 drops	12 drops	18 drops	30 drops	60 drops

Essential Oil Measurement Conversions

Drops	6	10	12	20	25	50	100
Milliliters	0.3	0.5	0.6	1	1.25	2.5	5
Teaspoons	–	–	⅛	–	¼	½	1

Chapter 11

Recipe Starters and Inspirations

Here you'll find thirteen recipe starters for common magickal practices, ready for your customization. Think of these as training wheels that will help you build knowledge, experience, and confidence in your custom blending.

For each recipe starter, I have provided essential oil suggestions for each magickal benefit and what I think might be a fitting method of use. You'll also notice that I included some visualization recommendations. These suggestions should help focus your intention for the magickal work and tap into the oils' boosting power. Use the recipes as guidelines—hopefully they empower you to get started and practicing in your unique way. When making them your own, take time to think about them, examine how they feel, and make changes that make sense to you. Use what works and change up what doesn't. Remember, the most important ingredient in any magickal recipe is you. My advice is to proceed with confidence and reverence when performing any spell or ritual.

When customizing these recipe starters, choose one essential oil per benefit. For example, to make the Clean AF blend, you would choose *either* lemon, tea tree, or peppermint essential oil to act as the "Cleanse" oil. Next, you would choose *either* frankincense, neroli, or clove bud essential oil to act as the "Infuse" oil. Finally, you would choose *either* rosemary, vetiver, or lemongrass essential oil to act as the "Protect" oil. Some of the recipe starters suggest a quantity, but remember that any aromatherapy blend can be scaled up or scaled down to suit your needs. Just pay attention to the ratio of essential oils to carrier (for safety), and determine the quantities of each essential oil based on your goals, subjective element, aroma, and dilution requirements. You've got this!

Clean AF Blend
100% Essential Oil

Just as we wouldn't prepare food in a dirty kitchen, spiritual work is best performed in an metaphysically clean environment. This pure essential oil blend is intended to be used to cleanse the energy of a space, infuse it with positive energy, and protect it from negativity and malevolence.

You will need

- 10 mL amber glass bottle
- An active diffuser, such as an ultrasonic or nebulizer

Essential oils

> *Cleanse:* lemon, tea tree, or peppermint
>
> *Infuse:* frankincense, neroli, or clove bud
>
> *Protect:* rosemary, vetiver, or lemongrass

Directions

1. Blend, as per your preferences, a total of up to 200 drops (2 teaspoons) to fill the 10 mL bottle.
2. Use the blend in an active diffuser to clean the energy and atmosphere of a room.
3. Use the blend as the key ingredient in a household surface cleaner (recipe below).

Visualization prompts for cleansing a space

The Cleanse oil pushes out and dissolves negative energies. You feel its clearing nature purifying your space.

The Infuse oil radiates with pure white light. This light holds the brightness of the sun, the warmth of joy, and the freedom of peace. Let it fill your space with bright blessings.

The Protect oil creates a barrier around your space. You set a strong boundary through which only love can cross.

May your space be cleansed and protected.

Clean AF Household Surface Cleaner Recipe

Of course, cleansing in the physical realm is also important for our overall well-being. In a physically clean space, people often find that they sleep better, think more clearly, and interact more harmoniously with others.

You will need

- Clean AF Blend—100% Essential Oil
- 16 oz. glass bottle with a spray mister top
- Measuring spoons
- Unscented castile soap
- Distilled water

Directions

1. In a 16 oz. glass bottle with a spray mister top, mix ⅓ teaspoon of the Clean AF blend into 2 tablespoons of unscented castile soap.
2. Fill the bottle to its shoulder with distilled water.
3. Shake before every use.

Ablution Blend
100% Essential Oil

This pre-ritual bathing blend is intended to cleanse and prepare the mind, body, and spirit for sacred work. It creates a sense of stillness and serenity that can be used to access higher realms of spiritual awareness.

You will need

- 10 mL amber glass bottle
- Unscented body wash (or castile soap)
- Small dish, like a ramekin, for use in the shower or bath.

Essential oils

Purify: juniper, lemon, or grapefruit

Refresh: Roman chamomile, rosemary, or peppermint

Restore: Australian sandalwood, frankincense, or sweet orange

Directions

1. Blend as per your preferences a total of up to 100 drops (1 teaspoon) to fill the 10 mL bottle.

2. Use by pouring about a teaspoon of bodywash into the small dish, then mixing in 3 drops of the Ablution blend. This makes a dilution of 3 percent essential oils in 97 percent bodywash.

3. Use to mindfully cleanse the body in the shower or bath before any sacred work.

Visualization prompts for cleansing the body in a pre-ritual bath or shower

The Purify oil draws out any toxic energies. Feel it pulling any negativity up and out, to be rinsed away.

The Refresh oil clears and fortifies your mind. You feel clear, peaceful, and focused.

The Restore oil fills any voids in your energy field with pure white light. It heals and rejuvenates you.

Let the water rinse away any unhelpful thoughts, feelings, and energies. You are cleansed and unburdened.

As you dry your blessed body, you feel ready for the sacred work to come. Let it begin!

Sacred Space and Meditation Blend
100% Essential Oils

This diffuser blend is intended to create a meditative atmosphere conducive to sacred work. It calms the mind, centers our energy, and makes it easier to connect with the divinity within and around us.

You will need

- 5 mL amber glass bottle
- An active diffuser, such as an ultrasonic or nebulizer

Essential oils

Ground: vetiver, patchouli, or myrrh

Prepare: Himalayan cedarwood, elemi, or frankincense

Connect: black spruce, cypress, or neroli

Directions

1. Blend as per your preferences a total of up to 100 drops (1 teaspoon) to fill the 10 mL bottle.
2. Actively diffuse into the environment for twenty minutes before or during your spiritual session.

Visualization prompts to ready the mind, body, and spirit for meditation and sacred work

Feel the energy of the Ground oil drawing down, anchoring you in your body. It brings a stillness that is supported and stable.

The Prepare oil brings you to center. You feel calm and balanced.

The Connect oil calls to the divine presence within and around you. You are a sacred being, empowered with healing purpose.

Earth Element Blend
3% Essential Oil in 97% Carrier Oil

The earth element anchors us to the physical realm and connects us to our bodies. It brings us the wisdom of lived experience drawn up from the soil. It is sure, steadfast, and solid. This blend is intended to call to the power of the earth.

You will need

- 30 mL amber glass bottle
- Olive oil

Essential oils

Health: copaiba, sage, or lavender

Soil: Australian sandalwood, vetiver, or patchouli

Truth: frankincense, rose, or black pepper

Directions

1. Blend as per your preferences a total of up to 18 drops of the Earth Element essential oils into the 30 mL bottle.

2. Use by adding 3 drops of the Earth Element blend to 1 teaspoon of olive oil (3% dilution).

3. To use, massage some of the blend into your lower body (legs, ankles, feet) while giving gratitude to all of the strong foundations that exist to support you.

Visualization prompts to connect
with the element of earth

Embody the stability of the olive tree and dig in your roots. You stand strong and feel at peace.

Sense the ancestral knowledge in the Soil oil and let it meld into your consciousness. You are grounded and supported.

Feel the oil of Health strengthening all the systems in your body. You are capable and full of vitality.

Listen to the oil of Truth acknowledging and honoring the incredible being that you are. You are confident and sure.

Attune to the powers of the earth element.

Air Element Blend

3% Essential Oil in 97% Water and Dispersant

The air element brings us clarity and connects us to the realm of the mind. It blows away what's no longer needed and creates space for expansion. It is quick, clarifying, and ever moving. This blend is intended to call to the element of air.

You will need

- 1 oz. amber glass bottle with a fine mist spray top
- Dispersant (e.g., polysorbate 20, solubol)
- Distilled water

Essential oils

> *Breeze:* eucalyptus, peppermint, or niaouli
>
> *Clear mind:* basil, frankincense, or rosemary
>
> *Conveyance:* lemon, German chamomile, or geranium

Directions

1. Pour the manufacturer recommended amount of your chosen dispersant into a 1 oz. glass bottle with a spray mister top.
2. Blend as per your preferences a total of 18 drops of essential oils to the dispersant and swirl to mix.
3. Fill the bottle with distilled water and shake before every use.
4. Use as a spray mist over and around your head.

Visualization prompts to connect with the element of air

Feel the cooling nature of the Breeze oil. Take in three refreshing breaths.

Sense how the Clear Mind oil loosens any mental blocks. Your thoughts and ideas flow freely.

The oil of Conveyance blows away mental fog and uncertainty. Your communication is crystal clear.

Attune to the powers of the air element.

Fire Element Blend
100% Essential Oil

The fire element is active and enthusiastic, but it also brings comfort as it draws us to the hearth. It fuels our courage and empowers us to be rid of what no longer serves us. It motivates and inspires us to act. This blend is intended to call to the element of fire.

You will need

- 5 mL amber glass bottle
- Tealight candles

Essential oils

Hearth: clove bud, black pepper, or cinnamon

Transformation: myrtle, mandarin, or ginger

Passion: cardamom, ylang-ylang, or petitgrain

Directions

1. Blend a total of up to 100 drops (1 teaspoon) in a 5 mL glass bottle.
2. Use with a tealight.
   a. Put 3 drops of the blend on top of the unlit tea candle. Light it and let it form a puddle of melted wax under the flame.
   b. Snuff out the flame and drop 1 or 2 drops of the essential oil blend into the melted wax

puddle. Relight the candle and let it burn. Be careful: the oil may cause the flame to sputter.

Visualization prompts to connect with the element of fire

The captivating flame emanating from the Hearth oil draws you in. Allow yourself to melt into the comfort of it.

Sense the emboldening nature of the Transformation oil. You can make the changes necessary to heal and transcend.

Feel the Passion oil activating your desires. You are fearless and eager.

Attune to the powers of the fire element.

Water Element Blend
100% Essential Oil

The Water element brings us all the feels! It's a life giver and deep healer that holds and nurtures us. As a shapeshifter that takes many forms, water reminds us that nothing is constant, and that change is good. This blend is intended to call to the element of Water.

You will need

- 5 mL amber glass bottle
- Bowl of warm water

Essential oils

> *Nurture:* German chamomile, jasmine, or rose
>
> *Emotions:* neroli, lavender, or bergamot
>
> *Intuition:* myrrh, black spruce, or yarrow

Directions

1. Blend as per your preferences a total of up to 100 drops (1 teaspoon) to fill the 5 mL bottle.
2. To use, add up to 10 drops total of essential oils into a dish of warm water. Let them passively diffuse into the environment.

Visualization prompts to connect with the element of water

Look into the dish of water and notice how the oils sit on its surface, supported by it, held by it. Take in the aroma.

Feel how the Nurture oil soothes and cares for you. You are reassured and calm.

Sense the healing nature of the Emotions oil bringing balance and perspective to your feelings. Your insight supports your mental wellness.

Hear your inner voice growing louder and clearer, heightened by the Intuition oil. You can trust your gut feelings.

Attune to the powers of the water element.

Spirit Element Blend
100% Essential Oil

The Spirit element is a divine unifier of enlightenment. Its omnipresence reminds us that we are never alone, and we're interconnected with all of Nature. It exists in and around all things, weaving us together in the beautiful tapestry of life and consciousness. This blend is intended to call to the element of spirit.

You will need

- 5 mL amber glass bottle
- Jojoba oil

  You: this can be anything that represents your unique magick

  Spiritual wellness: palmarosa, myrrh, or vetiver

  Divinity: frankincense, black spruce, or elemi

Directions

1. Blend as per your preferences a total of up to 100 drops (1 teaspoon) to fill the 5 mL bottle.

2. To use, actively diffuse into the environment. Alternatively, add 3 drops of the blend into 1 teaspoon jojoba oil. This makes a 3% dilution of essential oils in 97% jojoba oil to use topically as an anointing oil.

2b. Use this 3% dilution to anoint your body as a pentacle.

3. Use this 3 percent dilution to anoint your body as a pentacle: Visualize the star within a circle. To integrate yourself into this symbol of magick, anoint your third eye. Then draw a line of energy to your left ankle and anoint your left foot. Draw the energy to your right wrist and anoint your right hand. Repeat, next drawing to your left wrist, to your right ankle, and complete the pentacle star at your third eye.

Visualization prompts to connect with the element of spirit

Notice how the jojoba oil forms a protective barrier that is only penetrable by forms of love.

Feel the energy in the oil that represents you vibrating with magick. It awakens the spirit within and reminds you that the world needs your unique light.

Sense the balance of healing from the Spiritual Wellness oil. You are in harmony with the rhythm of the universe.

Connect to the oil of Divinity, resonating with the divine within and around you. You are in awe of the interconnectedness of all things.

Visualize the protective power of the pentacle integrated with your own. You stand exchanging energy with the pure white light of the Divine.

Attune to the element of spirit.

The Sun Blend
5% Essential Oil in 95% Water and Dispersant

The sun is a symbol of strength, courage, and success. It's a powerful motivator that commands the seasons, teaching us about the cycle of life, death, and rebirth. This blend is intended to honor and invoke the sun.

You will need

- 1 oz. amber glass bottle with a fine mist spray top
- Dispersant (e.g., polysorbate 20, solubol)
- Distilled water

Essential oils

Our great star: myrtle, lemon, or coriander seed

Expressiveness: neroli, scotch pine, or sweet orange

The annual cycle: helichrysum, patchouli, or
rosemary

Directions

1. Pour the manufacturer recommended amount of your chosen dispersant into a 1-ounce glass bottle that has a spray mister top.

2. Blend as per your preferences 30 drops of the essential oils into the dispersant and swirl to mix.

3. Fill the bottle to its shoulder with distilled water.

4. Shake before every use, and use as an atmosphere spray.

Visualization prompts to connect with the sun

The Great Star oil connects you to the life-giving sun. It draws down the sunlight, bathing you in its invigorating vitality.

Sense how the Expressiveness oil invites you step into the spotlight. You are confident and ready to let your inner light shine.

The Annual Cycle oil emanates resilience. It helps you thrive despite seasonal challenges. You are strong and supported, looking forward to each new day.

Attune to the sun.

The Full Moon Halo Blend
8% Essential Oil in 92% Grapeseed Oil

In command of the tides, the moon teaches us about the rhythm of ebb and flow, fullness, and release. The full moon could be compared to the moment of breath when we're at the capacity of an inhale, lungs full of air, ready to exhale. It is charged with active energy that illuminates our many blessings and encourages us to live a full life of meaningful experiences. This blend is intended to honor and invoke the full moon.

You will need

- 10 mL amber glass bottle with a roller-ball top
- Grapeseed oil

Essential oils

> *Silver light:* peppermint, clary sage, or ravintsara
>
> *Reflection:* jasmine, myrrh, or sweet fennel
>
> *Lunar cycle:* Australian sandalwood, rose, or frankincense

Directions

1. Blend as per your preferences a total of up to 16 drops in the roller top bottle.
2. Fill the bottle to its shoulder with grapeseed oil.
3. To use, apply this oil like a circlet around your head to create a moon halo. Starting at the center of your forehead, begin to apply a band that follows your hairline. Bring it along the side of your head, around to the back of your neck, around to the other side of your head, and back up to your third eye to complete the halo.

Visualization prompts to connect with the full moon

Feel the energy of abundance in the grapeseed oil.

The brightness of the moon shines as the oil of silver light. Draw it down and let it fill your entire being. You are truly blessed, and the universe is thankful that you are embracing your best life.

The Reflection oil invites you to look in the mirror of the moon. You see your purest self, luminous and beautiful, beaming light in all directions. Let your gratitude and love shine.

Connect to all the phases of the moon in the Lunar Cycle oil. Feel the balance and harmony. Take three deep, healing breaths. You are tapped into the wisdom of the universe, now and always.

Attune to the full moon.

The New Moon Halo Blend
9% Essential Oil in 91% Evening Primrose Oil

The new moon could be compared to the moment of breath when we're at the end of an exhale, lungs almost empty, getting ready to inhale.

You will need

- 10 mL amber glass bottle with a roller-ball top
- Evening primrose oil

Essential oils

Dark night: black spruce, patchouli, or sweet marjoram

Introspection: Roman chamomile, rose, or clary sage

Lunar cycle: Australian sandalwood, geranium, or melissa

Directions

1. Blend as per your preferences a total of up to 18 drops of essential oils in the roller top bottle.

2. Fill the bottle to its shoulder with evening primrose oil.

3. To use, apply this oil like a circlet around your head to create a moon halo. Starting at the center of your forehead, begin to apply a band that follows your hairline. Bring it along the side of your head, around to the back of your neck, around to the other side of your head, and back up to your third eye to complete the halo.

Visualization prompts to connect with the new moon

Feel how the evening primrose oil resonates with the mystery of the night.

Sense the tranquility of the moon in the Dark Night oil. Draw it down and let it quiet any chaos, bringing peace to your entire being. You are able to hear the whispers of the universe, guiding you toward the most beautiful blessings.

Feel how the oil of Introspection invites you to look within. You see your limitless potential and understand what needs to be done. Trust your intuition.

Connect to all the phases of the moon in the Lunar Cycle oil. Feel the balance and harmony. Take three deep, healing breaths. You are tapped into the wisdom of the Universe, now and always.

Attune to the new moon.

Consecration of Sacred Tools
10% Essential Oil in 90% Hemp Seed Oil

Our sacred tools often serve both a utilitarian and spiritual purpose. Through consecration, we can cleanse them of any residual energy they may carry and charge them with their magickal duties. In this process they become an extension of us, imbued with our energy and will. This blend is intended to facilitate the process of consecration, inviting divine guidance, protection, and personal power.

You will need

- 10 mL amber glass bottle
- Hemp seed oil

Essential oils

> *Divine touch:* cinnamon, lavender, or tea tree
> *Arcane knowledge:* sage, copaiba, or palmarosa
> *Power infusion:* basil, hyssop, or petitgrain

Directions

1. Blend as per your preferences a total of up to 20 drops in the 10 mL bottle.

2. Fill the bottle to its shoulder with hemp seed oil.

3. To use, apply a few drops of the Consecration blend to a soft cloth and gently polish your tool of magick, taking care to cover every surface. As you do so, envision the oil cleansing away any unwanted energy and saturating the tool with yours. Wipe off any excess oil so that your tool is not greasy.

Note: If the tool would be harmed or damaged by the application of oil, you can rub 10 drops into your hands and let it absorb into your skin. Instead of polishing, hold the tool in both hands and visualize the energy of each oil penetrating it, cleansing it, and charging it.

Visualization prompts for the consecration of sacred tools

Not only does the hemp oil imbue your tool with a spirit of generosity and abundance, it also offers an energy of practicality

As you hold your tool, feel the energy energy of the Divine Touch oil coursing through your hands and ordaining it as sacred, aligning it with your spiritual path.

The Arcane Knowledge oil transforms your tool into a vessel that will collect and hold ancient wisdom, providing you with profound spiritual guidance.

Channel your unique magick through the Power Infusion oil, charging it with your thoughts, dreams, plans, and all that is quintessentially you. This tool is yours, ready to be used in your spells, rituals, and all other forms of magick.

May your sacred tools serve to bring you, and others, all the bright blessings of the universe!

Divination Blend
6% Essential Oil in 94% Borage Oil

Divination can take many forms. The intention of this blend is to facilitate any kind of divination, from tarot reading to table-tipping. Use it to amplify your intuition, improve your psychic ability, and more effectively channel and communicate with divine entities.

You'll need

- 10 mL amber glass bottle
- Borage oil

Essential oils

Psychic boost: cannabis, cypress, or sweet fennel

Knowing: Himalayan cedarwood, coriander seed, or yarrow

Channel: Roman chamomile, bay leaf, or angelica root

Directions

1. Blend as per your preferences a total of up to 12 drops in the 10 mL bottle.
2. Fill the bottle to its shoulder with borage oil.
3. Using the visualization prompts below, apply the blend to your feet, solar plexus, hands, and third eye.

Visualization prompts to prepare for divination

First, apply this blend to your feet and ground yourself. Next, apply it to your stomach area, or wherever you physically sense your gut instincts. Feel the Knowing oil nurturing your intuition.

Now rub some into your hands. Hear the Channel oil calling to your divine guides, inviting them to join in the work ahead.

Finally, apply some over your third eye and establish a psychic barrier that will encourage communicative energy to be exchanged while protecting you from unwanted energies. The Psychic Boost oil amplifies your ability to tune into the subtle energies, screening out anything unwanted.

You are ready to safely receive messages from any divine beings who are invited and helpful. So be it!

Inspiration for Creating Custom Recipes

The following client vignettes showcase the flexibility of aromatherapy and magick. It's time to ditch the training wheels. As you start to venture into creating your own fully custom blends, I invite you to expand what you think is possible. The only rules (if they can be called that) are that magickal aromatherapy blends should contain oils with properties related to the intent of the ritual and each one should be crafted specifically to achieve your magickal goals. Let these stories offer creative inspiration for weaving the aromatic world of essential oils into your own spiritual practices and everyday life. As you begin to explore the possibilities for your aromatherapy and magick, don't hold yourself back—the sky is the limit!

Raphael, a Reiki master, has a practice that involves creating an energy grid using crystals and essential oils. They place crystals on the grid points and then use a dropper to carefully apply corresponding essential oils onto the crystals. For example, rose oil goes on the rose quartz, lavender oil goes on the amethyst crystal, and German chamomile oil on the turquoise stone. Raph experiences a deep sense of synergy when combining these three magickal healing modalities.

"Plant Whisperer" Petra is an avid gardener who works with the entity-like energies of plants. She uses a morning mist of clove and peppermint essential oils mixed with rainwater to spray around her garden while whispering positive affirmations. She finds that the essential oils act as a communication enhancer between her and the plants, helping them grow stronger and healthier.

Isabel, an intuitive artist, uses art as a form of spiritual expression. Before starting their painting sessions, they diffuse a blend of orange, ylang-ylang, and Australian sandalwood essential oils to stimulate their creativity and deepen their connection to the Divine. They notice that the aroma helps tap into deeper layers of their intuition, producing artwork that is both beautiful and spiritually meaningful.

Terrence is fascinated by the concept of past lives and time travel in the metaphysical sense. He has a meditation practice in which he uses certain oils to "travel" to different eras and dimensions. Cypress oil takes him to ancient Greece and myrrh oil to ancient Egypt. He applies these oils to his forehead and wrists (plus an anchoring oil to his feet) before starting his deep meditations.

Sylvie is a sound healer who combines the healing powers of sound bowls and essential oils in her practice. She places a few drops of essential oils, often eucalyptus or copaiba, into water before striking her crystal sound bowls. The vibration of the bowls disperses the aromatic molecules into the air, blending with the sound waves to create a unique multi-sensory healing experience.

Zara is a Zen Master who created an elaborate diffusion schedule to shift the energy at specific intervals during her meditation practice. Rather than diffusing the same essential oil throughout the entire length of a meditation, Zara starts with grounding vetiver, transitions to focusing rosemary, and then concludes with calming neroli.

Fiona is a Witch drawn to the realm of the Fae and other nature spirits. To communicate with them, she uses a blend of mandarin, Roman chamomile, and lavender essential oils. She anoints her garden statues and Faery altars with this blend, strengthening their connection.

By incorporating intentional aromatherapy, Mason transformed a mundane morning task into a spiritual practice. When preparing his daily caffeinated beverage, he mixes matcha powder with a drop of lemon and bergamot oils. He then whisks it in hot water and adds it to steamed oat milk. This infused latte brings an extra layer of mindfulness and alertness to the start of each day.

Celebrating the Wheel of the Year is an integral part of Dru's spiritual practice. For every seasonal holiday, he creates a magickal essential oil blend. His favorite day of celebration is Beltane, when he blends ylang-ylang, jasmine, and rose to honor fertility and love. He anoints himself and his ritual tools with this blend to imbue them with Beltane energy.

Tara is a tarot reader who uses angelica root essential oil to strengthen her readings and relationship with her cards. She puts a drop on her fingertips before shuffling her tarot deck. It helps her connect to her spirit guides, leading to clearer and more deeply understood card readings.

Chapter 12
Rad Recipes

In my opinion, part of being a Witch involves reimagining the world around us. I'm constantly seeing ways one could intertwine the mystical and mundane. The art of aromatherapy is an opportunity to innovate life's experiences. Picture this: aromatic bookmarks that release enchanting fragrance as you immerse yourself in a novel, lip balm that empowers its wearer to speak their truth, and stationery that sends aromatic letters of love. The realms of aromatherapy and magick are rife with opportunities to challenge boring old norms. This chapter offers ten of my favorite aromatherapy recipes with some less common magickal applications. I hope you'll find the process of crafting and concocting to be as rewarding as I do!

Rocket Fuel Ink

Even for skeptics who may not believe in the efficacy of magick, there can be no denying that symbols and words have power. Using infused ink for ritual use of iconography, symbology, and language might just become your newest standard magickal practice.

You'll need

- A dip pen
- Calligraphy ink for dip pens
- Dinky Dip jars with a base
- A dropper
- Essential oils of lime, basil, and lavender
- A 5 mL glass bottle with reducer cap or dropper
- A small funnel (optional, for adding the oils to the bottle)
- Watercolor paper (optional … but I love deckle edged, recycled cotton, watercolor paper for witchcraft)

Directions

1. In the 5 mL glass bottle, blend 60 drops of essential oils—17 drops basil, 20 drops lavender, and 23 drops lime. This will fill the bottle about ¾ full.

2. Take a dinky dip jar and add one drop of your essential oil blend.

3. Use the dropper to transfer some ink into that same dinky dip jar, close the lid tightly and shake to mix.

4. The ink is now charged with aromatherapy magick. Use your dip pen in this ink to draw sigils or write incantations for any spellcraft that you'd like to imbue with super lucky energy. Any paper should do, but my recommended paper is ideal.

5. When you have completed your ink work, dispose of the remaining ink in the dinky dip jar. Make a fresh batch for each new use.

Intention behind the oils

May the basil amplify the beautiful potential of your spellcraft. May the lavender attract supportive allies. May the lime start a wave of positive transformational energy. May you find yourself and your endeavors to be wildly successful!

Body Worship Lotion

I need you to listen to this with your entire being: You are fucking gorgeous. I mean, you are a legit powerhouse of beauty, sensuality, sexuality, and pure magick. Let this sink into your soul and register as a truth that you can trust, even if you can only believe me for a minute. Tomorrow, read this again. And the next day. And the next day. Keep trusting my words until you can see yourself how I see you.

You'll need

- Unscented body lotion
- Essential oils of marjoram, ylang-ylang, and patchouli
- A 5 mL glass bottle with reducer cap or dropper
- A small funnel (optional, for adding the oils to the bottle)

Directions

1. Combine your essential oils in the glass bottle—30 drops ylang-ylang, 20 drops marjoram, 5 drops patchouli. This will fill it about halfway.

2. Add 6 drops of the body worship blend into about a tablespoon of the unscented body lotion.

3. Visualize the body lotion transforming as it is filled with love, gratitude, admiration, and appreciation for your incredible body, and others.

4. Mix well and apply to skin.

Intention behind the oils

May the ylang-ylang bring you confidence. May the marjoram quiet your inner critic. May the patchouli connect you to the truth of your amazingness. May you worship your magickal body as often as possible!

A New Day Shower Tablets

Negative energies can be a bit sticky. Every morning we are given a new beginning, but sometimes it can be hard to wash off yesterday's energetic grime. Take one of these tablets and place it on the floor of your shower. When the hot water hits it, the room will fill with aromatherapy magick.

You'll need

- 1 cup baking soda
- ¾ cup cornstarch
- ½ cup of water
- Essential oils of rosemary and juniper
- A silicone muffin mold or ice cube tray
- Mixing bowl and a small bowl
- Measuring spoons and spatula
- A dropper
- A glass, airtight container for tablet storage

Directions

1. In the mixing bowl, combine the baking soda and cornstarch.

2. Add the water to the bowl, bit by bit. Slowly mix it into a clumping paste consistency, like magic mud.

3. Add ½ teaspoon of juniper essential oil and ½ teaspoon of rosemary essential oil and mix into the paste.

4. Put 1 to 2 tablespoons of the paste into each of the cups of your silicone mold. A tablet thickness of a ½ inch is ideal.

5. Preheat the oven to 350° F and bake for 15 to 20 minutes.

6. Remove and let them cool completely. They will continue to dry as they cool.

7. Blend ¼ teaspoon juniper and ¼ teaspoon rosemary in the small bowl and using the dropper, sprinkle the tablets with the essential oil blend. Let it soak into the hardening tablets then place them in your airtight glass container, for storage.

8. As you hop into your morning shower, simply toss a tablet onto the shower floor and enjoy.

Intention behind the oils

May the juniper detoxify your body and aura, leaving yesterday in the past. May the rosemary generate a shield of light, protecting you. May you feel refreshed, rejuvenated, and inspired to seize each new day.

Lucky Roller Perfume

Genuine effort is necessary to achieve our goals, but there are times when a little luck will take us a long way. Depending on the user and the context of their life, the lucky boost from this roller perfume will manifest in many wonderful and unexpected ways. It's safe to say that literally everything would benefit from what these oils bring! Wear this as an aromatherapy perfume with the intention to attract good fortune and to share its lucky magick everywhere you go.

You'll need

- A 10 mL glass bottle with a roller-ball top
- Sunflower oil
- Essential oils of bergamot, neroli, and helichrysum
- A small funnel (optional, for adding the oils to the bottle)

Directions

1. Blend the essential oils into the roller-ball bottle—10 drops bergamot, 7 drops neroli, and 3 drops helichrysum.

2. Add the sunflower oil to the bottle and fill it to its shoulder.

3. Pop in the roller-ball top and you have a 10% essential oil perfume blend ready to wear as a personal fragrance.

4. I also use it to draw little hearts and stars on random stuff in the world, including on telephone/ electricity poles, the back of park benches, city garbage cans, and trees.

Intention behind the oils

May the sunflower encourage your inner light to shine. May the bergamot lift any doubts. May the neroli attract incredible opportunities. May the helichrysum bring bright blessings. May we be able to see and celebrate all the luck we already benefit from and be ready for more!

Optimism and Momentum Lava Locket

This locket will serve well as a reminder to keep going, even when the going gets tough. Anytime you see or think of your locket, take a moment to breathe and take in its aroma. May the lava stone be the symbol of a clear path ahead.

You'll need

- An aromatherapy locket that holds a lava stone (could be on a keychain, a bracelet, etc.)

- Essential oils of orange, clary sage, and hyssop
- A 5 mL glass bottle with reducer cap or dropper
- A small funnel (optional, for adding the oils to the bottle)

Directions

1. Cleanse the lava stone and the locket by placing them in a bowl of salt overnight, then rinse with cold running water. Let them dry completely.

2. Place the locket in a sunny spot for a day so that it can absorb the sun's energy.

3. Combine equal parts of orange, clary sage, and hyssop essential oils in the bottle. I recommend 15 drops of each, which will only fill the bottle about halfway.

4. To "fill" the lava stone, place it in a small dish and carefully add a few drops of your essential oil blend directly onto the stone. Don't oversaturate it—just a few drops will do.

5. Once the lava stone has absorbed the oil, place it into the locket and securely close it. When you need to recharge the talisman, place it in the sunlight for a day before adding more of the essential oil blend.

Intention behind the oils

May the orange provide a boost of motivation. May the clary sage help you see how incredibly bright your future is. May the hyssop oil help you overcome any obstacles. May you move forward with ease and optimism.

Terracotta Protection Talisman

The desire for safety, well-being, and feeling in control over one's circumstances is a common human experience. Protection magick is a powerful way to both ward off potential harm and empower us to do what we can to stay safe.

> **One tip:** Although this talisman is intended to bring protection, it can be used to serve a broad spectrum of needs and preferences. Ultimately, it is a terracotta diffuser that can absorb any essential oil blend for aromatherapy magick.

You'll need

- Terracotta air dry clay, approx. 5oz
- A rolling pin
- Parchment baking paper to work on
- Essential oils of bay leaf, rosemary, and frankincense
- A small funnel (optional, for adding the oils to the bottle)

- A 10 mL glass bottle with a reducer cap or dropper
- A knife to cut clay
- A pentacle/pentagram cookie cutter
- A drinking straw or a clay cutting tool for holes
- 14-inch lengths of cord, string, or ribbon for hanging the talismans
- A plastic zip-top bag

Directions

1. Knead about 5 oz. of the terracotta air dry clay to soften it. This amount will make a few Terracotta Protection talismans.

2. On the parchment baking paper, roll out the clay to a thickness around ¼ inch.

3. Cut out pentacle shapes with your cookie cutter. Alternatively, you could use other cutter shapes, clay carvers, or patterned objects to press designs into the clay.

4. Use the end of the straw to cut a hole into the top of your clay shapes.

5. Let the clay shapes air dry for 48 hours. You might want to flip them at 24 hours so that they dry completely and evenly.

6. While the talismans are drying, blend the essential oils into the 10 mL glass bottle: ¼ teaspoon bay leaf, ¼ teaspoon frankincense, ¾ teaspoon

rosemary. This will fill the bottle a bit over halfway.

7. Once the talismans are fully dried, take a 14" length of cord, fold it in half, then thread the looped end through the hole on a clay pentagram talisman.

8. Tie a ring hitch knot to secure the cord to the talisman. Place your Terracotta talisman in some sunlight for a day to charge it, then as the sun sets, place it into the plastic bag and seal it to protect the talisman from moisture. Set it overnight under the moonlight to charge it for a second time, balancing the sun and moon energy within it.

9. Add up to 5 drops of your essential oil blend to the back of the talisman. The essential oil blend will slowly evaporate, passively diffusing into the environment. Hang it from a tree bough, a car rearview mirror, a doorknob, or wear it around your neck—wherever you feel needs it. When the aroma fades, just add more essential oil.

Intention behind the oils

May the terracotta embody the stability of Earth. May the rosemary bring alert awareness of surroundings. May the bay leaf be a shield against injury. May the frankincense call to the Divine to stand guard, protecting your good health. May you and yours be safe, always.

Blessed Bubbles

The need for healing in our world is both urgent and great. It requires a multidimensional approach that addresses root causes and not just the symptoms of the global ailments we face. It's complex and I don't know the solutions, but I do know that only through cooperative, holistic, and ongoing approaches can we even hope to heal our world … and more bubbles will definitely help.

You'll need

- ¼ teaspoon guar gum
- ½ teaspoon baking powder
- ½ tablespoon rubbing alcohol
- 2¼ tablespoon unscented dish soap (I really like Dawn)
- 2½ cups warm distilled water
- Essential oils of bergamot, grapefruit, rose, myrrh, and Australian sandalwood
- A mixing bowl
- A large glass jar
- Bubble wands

Directions

1. Put the warm water into your jar.
2. In the mixing bowl combine the guar gum and rubbing alcohol until it is a smooth and consistent liquid. Then add 1 drop of each essential oil into it, for a total of 5 drops.
3. Start to stir the water in the jar and pour the guar gum mixture into the moving water.
4. Still stirring, add in the dish soap followed by the baking powder.
5. Put the lid on your jar of magickal bubble juice and let it rest for 24 hours. After it has rested, it's ready to blow!

Intention behind the oils

May the bergamot spread true joy. May the grapefruit bring healthy abundance. May the rose invoke the power of love. May the myrrh ensure justice. May the sandalwood foster peace and compassion. May these blessed bubbles float out into the world and contribute to a more harmonious and sustainable future.

Heal Thyself Simmer Pot

Maintaining a home that supports whole health is crucial for overall well-being. It's a blessing that ripples out into all aspects of our lives. Although fine for every season, this recipe is particularly great in the fall and winter when our immune systems tend to be most challenged.

You'll need

- A medium sized pot (6 cup capacity)
- Essential oils of clove bud, orange, lemon, cinnamon, eucalyptus, and rosemary
- A 5 mL glass bottle with a reducer cap or dropper
- A small funnel (optional, for adding the oils to the bottle)
- Dried whole cloves, cinnamon sticks, rosemary sprigs, eucalyptus twig, lemon and orange peel (optional, but they look beautiful in the simmer pot)

Directions

1. Combine the essential oils in the 5 mL bottle—20 drops clove bud, 10 drops cinnamon, 10 drops lemon, 8 drops orange, 8 drops eucalyptus, 5 drops rosemary. This will fill the bottle just over halfway.

2. Pour about 4 cups of water into your pot and add the plant matter. Again, the sticks and leaves and peels are optional, but they really add to the whole experience.

3. Drip 4 drops of your essential oil blend into the filled pot. If you are not including plant matter, use 5 or 6 drops of the blend.

4. Put the filled pot onto the stove element and heat on a low temperature setting.

5. Let the pot simmer for about 30 minutes, adding water as needed. Limit simmer sessions to twice per day, maximum.

Intention behind the oils

May the clove bring warmth and the cinnamon bring comfort. May the freshness of the lemon clear the air. May the orange invoke the sun, flooding your space with healing light. May the eucalyptus and rosemary promote and protect the health of your home and body. May this powerhouse blend kill off any viruses or bad bacteria that threaten your well-being.

Dreamwork Pillow

Our dreams offer access to a realm where anything is possible. Dreamwork helps us process our inner worlds and explore other dimensions of reality. Before sleeping, take a moment to hold your Dreamwork pillow close. Breathe deeply, inhaling the gentle scents, and set an intention for your dreamscape. Pop it into, or under your regular pillow and sleep well.

You'll need

- Dark-colored natural fabric, such as cotton or silk, cut into two rectangles (approx. 12 x 6 inches each)
- Sewing needle and thread
- Dried lavender blossoms plus dried beans or rice to fill the pillow
- Essential oils of palmarosa, vetiver, patchouli, German chamomile
- Two bowls, one medium and one small
- A dropper
- Cotton balls
- A plastic zip-top bag

Directions

1. Place the two pieces of fabric together, with the right-sides in, facing each other. The right side of fabric is the side you want showing on your finished pillow.
2. Sew along three of the edges, leaving one short edge open.
3. After sewing, turn the fabric right-side out. You've made a pillow casing, yay!
4. In the medium bowl, combine the dried lavender and beans (or whatever fillings you choose).

5. Blend your essential oils in the small bowl: 4 drops palmarosa, 2 drops vetiver, 3 drops patchouli, 3 drops German chamomile.

6. Drop two cotton balls into the bowl so they can soak up the essential oil blend.

7. Loosely fill about ⅓ of the pillow by adding a layer of rice and lavender. Then add a soaked cotton ball.

8. Continue filling with another ⅓ layer of rice and lavender, add another soaked cotton ball. The pillow will be about half full at this point.

9. Add the final ⅓ of the filling mixture into the pillow. Adjust the pillow's firmness/flexibility by adding a bit more filling or by removing some.

10. Sew the open edge to close the pillow.

11. Place your Dreamwork pillow into the zip-top bag and seal it to protect it from moisture. Then set it outside under the moonlight to charge overnight.

12. When it no longer serves its purpose, I suggest composting it. Instead of recharging this pillow, just make a new one.

Intention behind the oils

May the palmarosa calm your nerves and bring relaxation. May the soothing patchouli help your body melt into the comfort of your bed. May the German chamomile rock you gently to sleep. May the vetiver serve as an anchor and map that will help you navigate the dream space. May the dried lavender bring whole healing. May your dreamwork be insightful and enriching!

Travel and Discovery Vial

Travel and discovery are as much about the internal world as they are about the external world. This vial acts as a reminder to live in the present and experience all that we can in the now. Whether walking around your neighborhood or flying across the sea, every day offers opportunities for learning, change, and expansion through exploration.

You'll need

- A small glass vial with a cork stopper or screw cap
- Black tourmaline fragments (small enough to fit in the vial)
- A small funnel (optional, for adding the stones and oils to the vial)
- Essential oils of grapefruit, angelica root, and ylang-ylang
- A small bowl and a dropper
- A strong, thin piece of cord or chain (optional, to wear the vial as a necklace or bracelet)
- Super glue or sealing wax

Directions

Before you put the black tourmaline into the vial, cleanse it by leaving it in a bowl of salt overnight, then rinsing with cold running water. Leave to dry.

1. Use a small funnel (or your fingers) to place some black tourmaline fragments inside the vial.

2. Combine equal parts of essential oils in a small bowl. The combined amount depends on the size of the vial. With the stones inside, the oil blend should almost fill it.

3. Use a dropper to fill the vial up to its shoulder with the essential oil blend. Do not fill the vial all the way up to the top, especially if you will be closing it with a cork.

4. Screw on cap or place the cork to close the vial. Seal it closed with wax or a bit of super glue. If desired, attach a cord or chain.

5. Leave the vial overnight in a place where it can absorb the moonlight.

6. Carry the vial with you as you adventure through your incredible life. Before heading out into the world, hold the vial in your hands and use it as a tangible reminder to be present.

Intention behind the oils

May the black tourmaline keep you from harm. May the grapefruit oil invite unexpected delights. May the angelica keep your guardians close. May the ylang-ylang bring fun adventures. May your journey be blessed!

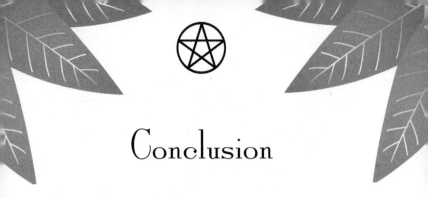

Conclusion

This book represents the core principles and processes of my approach to aromatherapy and magick. It's an expression of my knowledge and experience, but it's ultimately about you. The more you use essential oils in your spiritual practices, the stronger your relationships with them become. As your relationships grow stronger, so do the energy exchanges. When the intensity of the energy exchanges is increased, so are the linked magickal smell memories. Our magickal smell memories from yesterday add power to our spiritual practices today. Naturally, our spiritual practices will therefore incorporate essential oils more and more often … and the cycle of healing continues in an upward spiral of expansion and growth.

I hope that this book serves as a guiding light on that path, illuminating the transformative power of aromatherapy in magickal practices, promoting wellness on all levels, and fostering deeper, more enriched spiritual experiences. It is an invitation to explore, understand, and embrace the beautiful complexity of essential oils as we build harmonious relationships with them. Their non-judgmental and direct healing nature makes them steadfast friends on our spiritual journeys, always inviting us to further discover the magick within and around us.

A journey with aromatherapy and magick is not just a journey of personal enlightenment and wellness but also one of responsibility. As conscientious citizens of our planet, our choices—particularly about essential oils—reflect our commitment to both whole health and environmental stewardship. We can't really make wrong choices in this endeavor because the ultimate goal is to seek a better path that also resonates with our individual beliefs, experiences, and needs.

As we draw this to a close, reflect upon what you've uncovered. What have you learned about yourself and your beliefs? How have you grown? Where do you want to go from here? The way ahead is laden with treasures—all you need to do is seek them out. As you move forward on your sacred journey, let your intuition be your compass, the oils your allies, and your uniqueness a scythe that cuts a new path. May you find healing, inspiration, and love in a universe teeming with possibilities and limitless magick. In deep gratitude, so mote it be!

Special Thanks

First off, this book would not exist without Heather Greene's encouragement. Thank you, Heather, for your patience and inspiration.

Special thanks to Chrissy Ludmila for drawing the beautiful illustrations in this book. Chrissy, your willingness of spirit and generosity of time means the world.

To all you readers, you have my deepest gratitude. May the future bring all the blessings to fulfill your biggest dreams. So be it!

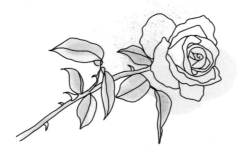

Recommended Reading

Adler, Margot. *Drawing Down the Moon: Witches, Druids, Goddess-Worshippers, and Other Pagans in America.* Penguin Books, 1997.

Auryn, Mat. *Psychic Witch: A Metaphysical Guide to Meditation, Magick & Manifestation.* Llewellyn Publications, 2020.

Ballard, H. Byron. *Roots, Branches & Spirits: The Folkways & Witchery of Appalachia.* Llewellyn Publications, 2021.

Beachy, Jenya T. *The Secret Country of Yourself: Discover the Powerful Magic of Your Endless Inner World.* Llewellyn Publications, 2017.

Berwick, Ann. *Aromatherapy: A Holistic Guide: Balancing Body and Soul with Essential Oils.* Llewellyn Publications, 1994.

Beyerl, Paul V. *The Master Book of Herbalism.* Phoenix Publishing Inc., 1984.

Billington, Penny. *The Path of Druidry: Walking the Ancient Green Way*. Llewellyn Publications, 2011.

Blackthorn, Amy. *Blackthorn's Botanical Magic: The Green Witch's Guide to Essential Oils for Spellcraft, Ritual & Healing*. Weiser Books, 2018.

Blanton, Crystal, Taylor Ellwood, Brandy Williams, eds. *Bringing Race to the Table: Exploring Racism in the Pagan Community*. Megalithica Books. 2015.

Buckland, Raymond. *Buckland's Complete Book of Witchcraft*. Llewellyn Publications, 2017.

Butje, Andrea. *The Heart of Aromatherapy: An Easy-to-Use-Guide for Essential Oils*. Hay House Inc, 2017.

Catty, Suzanne. *Hydrosols: The Next Aromatherapy*. Healing Arts Press, 2001.

Chen, Pamela. *Enchanted Crystal Magic: Spells, Grids & Potions to Manifest Your Desires*. Llewellyn Publications, 2021.

Granddaughter Crow. *Wisdom of the Natural World: Spiritual and Practical Teachings from Plants, Animals & Mother Earth*. Llewellyn Publications, 2021.

Cunningham, Scott. *The Complete Book of Incense, Oils and Brews*. Llewellyn Publications, 2002.

———. *Cunningham's Encyclopedia of Magical Herbs*. Llewellyn Publications, 1985.

———. *Magical Aromatherapy: The Power of Scent*. Llewellyn Publications, 1989.

———. *Magical Herbalism: The Secret Craft of the Wise.* Llewellyn Publications, 1986.

———. *Wicca: A Guide for the Solitary Practitioner.* Llewellyn Publications, 1989.

Davis, Patricia. *Aromatherapy An A-Z: The Most Comprehensive Guide to Aromatherapy Ever Published.* Vermilion, 2005.

———. Astrological Aromatherapy. Random House UK, 2002.

———. *Subtle Aromatherapy.* Random House UK, 1996.

Dorsey, Lilith. *Orishas, Goddesses and Voodoo Queens: The Divine Feminine in the African Religious Traditions.* Weiser Books, 2020.

Dulsky, Danielle. *The Holy Wild: A Heathen Bible for the Untamed Woman.* New World Library, 2018.

Farrar, Janet, and Stuart Farrar. *A Witches' Bible.* Phoenix Publishing, 1996.

———. *The Witches' God.* Phoenix Publishing, 1989

———. *The Witches' Goddess.* Phoenix Publishing, 1987.

Foxwood, Orion. *Mountain Conjure and Southern Root Work.* Weiser Books, 2021.

Gattefossé, Renee-Maurice. *Gattefossé's Aromatherapy: The First Book on Aromatherapy,* translated from French by Robert B. Tisserand. CW Daniels UK, 1996.

Heldstab, Celeste Rayne. *Llewellyn's Complete Formulary of Magical Oils: Over 1200 Recipes, Potions & Tinctures for Everyday Use*. Llewellyn Publications, 2012.

Higginbotham, River, and Joyce Higginbotham. *Paganism: An Introduction to Earth-Centered Religions*. Llewellyn Publications, 2002.

His Holiness the Dalai Lama. *The Universe in a Single Atom: The Convergence of Science and Spirituality*. Morgan Road Books, 2005.

Hughes, Kristoffer. *From the Cauldron Born: Exploring the Magic of Welsh Legend & Lore*. Llewellyn Publications, 2012.

Hutton, Ronald. *The Triumph of the Moon: A History of Modern Pagan Witchcraft*. Oxford University Press, 2001.

K, Amber. *True Magick: A Beginner's Guide*. Llewellyn Publications, 1990.

Kynes, Sandra. *Mixing Essential Oils for Magic: Aromatic Alchemy for Personal Blends*. Llewellyn Publications, 2013.

Lawless, Julia. *Aromatherapy and the Mind*. Thorsons, 1994.

———. *The Encyclopedia of Essential Oils: The Complete Guide to the Use of Aromatic Oils in Aromatherapy, Herbalism, Health & Well-Being*. Thorson Element, 1992.

LeFae, Phoenix. *What is Remembered Lives: Developing Relationships with Deities, Ancestors & the Fae.* Llewellyn Publications, 2019.

Lief, Judith L. *Making Friends with Death: A Buddhist Guide to Encountering Mortality.* Shambala Publications, 2001.

Lipton, Bruce H. *The Biology of Belief: Unleashing the Power of Consciousness, Matter, & Miracles.* Hay House, 2008.

Mankey, Jason. *Witch's Wheel of the Year: Rituals for Circles, Solitaries & Covens.* Llewellyn Publications, 2019.

Minetor, Randi. *Essential Oils of the Bible: Connecting God's Word to Natural Healing.* Althea Press, 2016.

Mojay, Gabriel. *Aromatherapy for Healing the Spirit: Restoring Emotional and Mental Balance with Essential Oils.* Henry Holt & Company, 1996.

Mooney, Thorn. *The Witch's Path: Advancing Your Craft at Every Level.* Llewellyn Publications, 2021.

Moura, Ann. *Green Witchcraft: Folk Magic, Fairy Lore & Herb Craft.* Llewellyn Publications, 2002.

———. *Origins of Modern Witchcraft: The Evolution of a World Religion.* Llewellyn Publications, 2000.

Pamita, Madame. *The Book of Candle Magic: Candle Spell Secrets to Change Your Life.* Llewellyn Publications, 2020.

Penczak, Christopher. *The Outer Temple of Witchcraft: Circles, Spells, and Rituals.* Llewellyn Publications, 2004.

Rose, Jeanne. *The Aromatherapy Book: Applications & Inhalations.* North Atlantic Books, 1993.

Starhawk. *The Earth Path: Grounding Your Spirit in the Rhythms of Nature.* HarperCollins, 2004.

———. *The Spiral Dance: A Rebirth of the Ancient Religion of the Great Goddess.* HarperOne, 1999. Originally published 1979 by Harper & Row.

Taylor, Astrea. *Intuitive Witchcraft: How to Use Intuition to Elevate Your Craft.* Llewellyn Publications, 2020.

Tisserand, Robert B. *The Art of Aromatherapy: The Healing and Beautifying Properties of the Essential Oils of Flowers and Herbs.* Healing Arts Press, 1978.

Wilson, Roberta. *Aromatherapy for Vibrant Health & Beauty.* Avery, 1995.

Worwood, Valerie Ann. *Aromatherapy for the Soul: Healing the Spirit with Fragrance and Essential Oils.* New World Library, 2006.

———. *The Complete Book of Essential Oils and Aromatherapy.* New World Library, 2016.

Zakroff, Laura Tempest, and Jason Mankey. *The Witch's Altar: The Craft, Lore & Magick of Sacred Space.* Llewellyn Publications, 2018.

Bibliography

Bagetta, Giacinto, Marco Cosentino, and Tsukasa Sakurada. *Aromatherapy: Basic Mechanisms and Evidence Based Clinical Use.* CRC Press, 2015.

Osbaldeston, Tess Anne, and Robert P. A. Wood. *Dioscorides: De Materia Medica: A New Indexed Version in Modern English.* IBIDIS Press, 2000.

Rocke, A. J. "Agricola, Paracelsus, and 'Chymia.'" *Ambix* 32, no. 1, (1985): 38–45.

Watson, Gerard. "Aristotle's Concept of Matter." *Philosophical Studies* 20 (1971): 175–84.

Index

To Write to the Author

If you wish to contact the author or would like more information about this book, please write to the author in care of Llewellyn Worldwide Ltd. and we will forward your request. Both the author and publisher appreciate hearing from you and learning of your enjoyment of this book and how it has helped you. Llewellyn Worldwide Ltd. cannot guarantee that every letter written to the author can be answered, but all will be forwarded. Please write to:

Dree Amandi Pike
⅗ Llewellyn Worldwide
2143 Wooddale Drive
Woodbury, MN 55125-2989

Please enclose a self-addressed stamped envelope for reply, or $1.00 to cover costs. If outside the U.S.A., enclose an international postal reply coupon.

Many of Llewellyn's authors have websites with additional information and resources. For more information, please visit our website at http://www.llewellyn.com.